Breeding Better
· ·
Vermonters

Revisiting New England: The New Regionalism

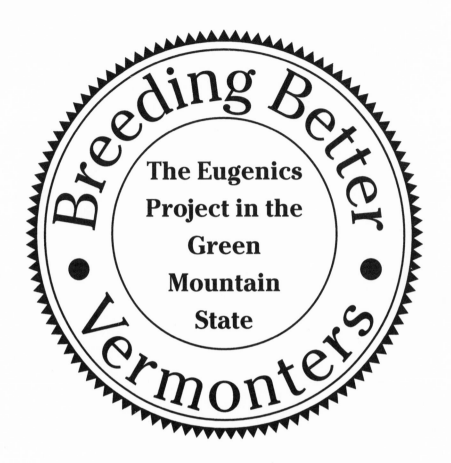

Breeding Better Vermonters

The Eugenics Project in the Green Mountain State

Nancy L. Gallagher

University Press of New England

HANOVER AND LONDON

University Press of New England, Hanover, NH 03755

© 1999 by Nancy L. Gallagher

All rights reserved

Printed in the United States of America

5 4 3 2 1

CIP data appear at the end of the book

To

CONNIE GALLAGHER,

who encouraged me to ask historical questions

and who taught me how little our biology

has to do with our humanity.

Contents

Illustrations

Preface

I first became acquainted with the Eugenics Survey of Vermont ten years ago during interdisciplinary projects with my biology students concerning bioethics, science and society issues, and historical controversies over biological theories. Eugenics inevitably surfaces in such projects, but at that time I took comfort in the prevailing orthodoxy that eugenics had more to do with politics and social history than with the subject I taught. But I soon came to learn the artificiality of such distinctions, as my inclusion in science class of such topics as birth control, medical genetics, and world population problems fell under the scrutiny of religious conservatives, who saw such teaching as "secular humanism," a form of child abuse in scientific and academic disguise. I became more interested in the history of biology and its human applications, particularly the fragile and permeable boundaries between science, politics, and religion that had dissolved in my own science classroom.

When I took up Vermont Eugenics as a thesis project, I intended to make a case study of how the Eugenics Survey functioned to promote biological perspectives on human problems through placing them within a familiar cultural framework. What began as a personal pilgrimage into the history of the science I had taught for twenty years became a deeper inquiry into the penetration and persistence of eugenic ideas and controversies in twentieth-century discourse on family life, health care, and social welfare problems. My research coincided with a surge of publicity on the Eugenics Survey of Vermont in art, journalism, and politics. Themes of conspiracy and concealment, Nazi connections, and racial purification were dramatized by portraying the Eugenics Survey as a repressed state scandal. Many were shocked to hear that "eugenics" happened "*even* in Vermont." Debates erupted over whether Vermont author Dorothy Canfield Fisher, who served with Eugenics Survey of Vermont Director Harry Perkins on the Vermont Commission on Country Life, was really a eugenicist (how could she be, when she wrote a book condemning anti-Semitism?). UVM students reported in history classes that the Nazis trained for eugenics in Vermont. Rumors still surface on campus of zoology professor Harry Perkins's systematic rounding up and sterilization of Native American, African American, and French Canadian Vermonters.

While these caricatures of eugenics have sensitized us to our racist past, they have also kept discussions of Vermont eugenics in a historiographical backwater, ensconced in the convenient labels of pseudoscience or racism, or viewed as precedents for genocide and thus further alienated from our values and experience. Consequently, there has been precious little discussion of Vermont's past eugenics ventures during deliberations on the new "Vermont Human Genetics Initiative," a program to integrate medical genetics into the state health care system, or the 1998 law authorizing the creation of a state DNA bank of blood samples of all persons convicted of a violent crime. While early detection and mandatory reporting of symptoms of mental instability, child abuse, or high risk behaviors among Vermont youth has intensified, little notice has been taken of the historical connection between the current infatuation with "prevention and intervention" and their precedents in the eugenics era. The most frequent reaction I have encountered to my work on this subject is, "What is eugenics and what does it have to do with us?" It seemed to me that our discussions of eugenics history, its meaning, and its largely unconscious legacy might benefit from a better understanding of the man and the enterprise behind the legend, particularly who studied whom, for what purpose, and with what results. This book is one contribution to what I hope will be a larger inquiry into this important chapter in our past, a past which is still deeply resonant for many people today.

Acknowledgments

My research and writing on eugenics was enriched by many people who enlarged my perspective, offered new insights, and supported my efforts. This book would never have been possible without the counsel and enthusiastic support of my advisor and editor, Dr. Dona Brown, who helped me to maintain the balance between historical perspective and creative license. Holocaust historian Doris Bergen provided valuable criticism and gave me the courage to confront the injustices in my own culture as well as a commitment to seek historical understanding of them. I wish to thank Professor Robert Gordon of the University of Vermont and Professor Jere Daniell of Dartmouth College, who critically reviewed my work and made important suggestions.

I benefited from the interest, recollections, and perspectives offered by T. D. Seymour Bassett and Irving Lisman, who gave me a sense of the context and personalities of those involved in the Eugenics Survey and suggestions for improving the manuscript. I am indebted to Samuel B. Hand, whose philosophical insights into Vermont history, as revealed in Vermont sources and government documents, provided the initial inspiration for my work, and to Kevin Dann, whose original research on Vermont eugenics raised the questions and provided many sources that served as the starting point for my own inquiry.

My research coincided with a resurgence of public interest in Vermont eugenics sparked by Michael Oatman's exhibit, "Long Shadows," at the Robert Hull Fleming Museum. I wish to thank Michael Oatman and Janie Cohen for including me in the lectures and forums associated with it. The eugenics artifacts that Michael discovered enriched my own research, and his show brought me in contact with many people who shared their memories, their research, their diverse perspectives, and the ways in which eugenics history was connected to their lives. From these interactions, I came to understand the importance of writing eugenics history into Vermont history. I would like to thank John Moody, Donna Roberts, and members of the Abenaki community, who helped me to develop a deeper sensitivity to the families in the survey records and an awareness of the meaning of Vermont eugenics to the history of native peoples.

My research benefited from the generous assistance of librarians, historians, and archivists. I wish to thank Connell Gallagher, Jeffrey Marshall, and the Special Collections faculty and staff at the Bailey Howe Library at the University of Vermont for their interest, service, and permission to publish materials in their collections and Roger Weiberg for his help in preparing visuals. I am grateful for the generous assistance of Clayton Marshia and John Yacavoni at the Vermont Public Records Office, who facilitated my work with the Eugenics Survey archive. My understanding of the Eugenics Survey collection was enhanced by my participation in a grant from the Vermont Historical Records Advisory Board to survey the Eugenics Survey archives. I am especially grateful for their support. I would like to thank the Vermont Children's Aid Society and the manuscripts librarians at Yale University Library and the American Philosophical Society for providing me with important source material and granting me permission to publish material from their collections.

This study has been profoundly influenced by my own students and colleagues and by the families in Vermont communities where I taught science for many years. As I pursued my research, I recalled many experiences in which Vermonters continue to suffer the indignity of policies based on false perceptions and judgments of their worth from superficial indicators. Poignant memories of their struggles provided the human faces that informed this study and urged me to complete it. Eugenics also forces us to think about the meaning of family. Throughout this project I became especially aware of how my own family, through their love, patience, and experience provided my center and my source of commitment to seeking the truth behind the facts.

March 1999   N.L.G.

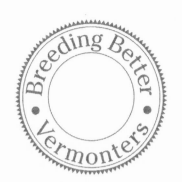

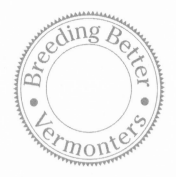

Introduction

> "When *I* use a word," Humpty Dumpty said, in a rather scornful tone, "it means just what I choose it to mean—neither more nor less."
>
> "The question is," said Alice, "whether you *can* make words mean different things."
>
> "The question is," said Humpty Dumpty, "which is to be master—that's all."
>
> **—Lewis Carroll, *Through the Looking Glass***

Eugenics means different things to different people. Francis Galton, the Victorian aristocrat and nephew of Charles Darwin, invented the term, meaning "well-born," in the 1880s. Galton believed that the key to human progress would rest on a national program of better breeding, in which the intelligent and the accomplished, the men and women of demonstrated high moral character—the educated upper classes—would conceive more children, while the shiftless, the chronic poor, the insane and feebleminded, and the "criminal class" would be discouraged, preferably prevented, from breeding at all. Over time, Galton predicted, the former would dominate the latter, and the "English race" would be strengthened physically, intellectually, and morally. Galton's ideas grew in popularity after 1900 as he and other scientists offered their revelations of the biological, mathematical laws governing heredity as the means by which human social progress might be informed and directed by science, not philosophy or religion. Galton's 1904 definition of eugenics became the official one for the twentieth century: "The study of agencies un-

1

der social control that may improve or impair the racial qualities of future generations, either physically or mentally." The focus on race, social control, and genetic "improvement," while inspiring pioneering studies in human genetics, also became a social weapon.

"Indeed, eugenics was conceived by its founders as a way of lifting humans toward greater perfection," biologist Ernst Mayr lamented in his 1984 essay, "The Origin of Human Ethics." "It is sadly ironic that this noble original objective eventually led to some of the most heinous crimes mankind has ever seen."[1] Evidently the line between good intentions and malice aforethought is a fine one. As Galton's "noble vision" inspired an international, interdisciplinary movement of scholars, scientists, medical experts, wealthy philanthropists, and government leaders eager to apply the new research, the eugenic solutions offered—mental testing, segregation and sterilization of the "unfit," marriage restrictions, and discriminatory immigration quotas—turned eugenics history into something of a no-man's-land of betrayal of trust, loss of privacy and freedom, broken families and broken lives. When the Third Reich translated eugenics into a program of racial purification through genocide, the Holocaust came to epitomize, for many people, the purpose, character, and meaning of eugenics.

Since World War II, the eugenics movement has provided historians with fertile territory for study of the dynamic interface between science, culture, and politics. The first histories of the eugenics movement, written during the civil rights era, emphasized the racist and pseudoscientific character of eugenics and made heroes of its critics. The past decade of historical research on eugenics has broadened our understanding of the eugenics movement to reveal its complexity, its continuity in present genetics and social research programs, and its ambiguous and changing role in the history of modern biological thought. "Eugenics" thus eludes any simple definition. The eugenics movement was international, politically diverse, and wrought with internal tensions as its moral and scientific ambiguities became apparent. As Martin Pernick notes, "Like such turn-of-the-century catchwords as *progressivism* and *efficiency*, the term *eugenics* encompassed a large and shifting constellation of meanings." In addition, criticism of eugenics (both scientific and ethical) was less rooted in scientific knowledge or in altruism than we have been led to believe. A variety of case studies and local studies have demonstrated how eugenics ideas and methods were adapted to different purposes and succeeded or failed depending on how effectively they were promoted within particular political or social cultures.[2]

Despite its heterogeneity, the eugenics movement provided a unifying paradigm, common themes, and a new language of biological determinism that gained strong support during the first three decades of the twentieth century, as new research programs in human heredity promised to provide a more scientific approach to ensuring the national health, preventing crime and poverty, and preserving the national character. Eugenics provided intellectuals in many fields with an interdisciplinary forum to apply their research to the common goal of human betterment. It appealed to progressive intellectuals' faith in science as the means to solve human problems, their trust in professional experts to provide reliable information, and their infatuation with cause and prevention, rather than cure or treatment, of human social and health problems. The eugenics movement, led in America by biologists who embraced Mendelian genetics, attracted a broad and powerful constituency and generated a vast literature that influenced public policy concerning immigration, mental health initiatives, and state intervention in family life.

Eugenicists promoted the idea that the *human germplasm* was the most important thing in the world, the source of all human potential in a nation or race. As such, it demanded cultivation and conservation. The handicapped, the mentally incompetent, and the chronic dependents on poor relief compromised, in the eugenicists' view, the future of the human race by contributing their genes too liberally to the national germplasm through indiscriminate breeding and having too many "unwanted children." Likewise, the highly educated upper classes and the "old pioneer stocks" in particular were blamed for what Theodore Roosevelt called "race suicide" in their trend toward smaller families. Believing that scientific knowledge of human heredity should inform public policy and that an individual's reproductive behavior was a matter of public interest, eugenicists embarked on propaganda campaigns to cultivate public awareness of the importance of eugenic breeding and to garner public support for eugenics legislation. Modern societies, they argued, required persons of higher intelligence, physical constitution, adaptability, and social instincts. The growing population of patients in state hospitals for the insane and special schools for the "feebleminded" provided researchers with defined populations on which to conduct studies demonstrating the inheritance of feeblemindedness, insanity, and asocial behavior. Statistics on the rising numbers of dependents—paupers, criminals, feebleminded, and the mentally ill—were cited as evidence of a growing threat to the nation's health and prosperity. When the public expense of target populations was linked to their birthrates, procreation became a public issue. In both England and the United States such studies fed anxieties that the population was deteriorating physically and mentally due to the unrestricted reproduction of genetically inferior persons. Marriage restrictions, segregation in institutions, and sterilization laws (negative eugenics measures) dramatically affected the lives of the people who were investigated eugenically. Less tangible, but more powerful perhaps, was the rhetoric of degeneracy that the eugenics studies introduced, which validated long-held prejudices and encouraged discrimination.

Eugenics attracted substantial funding for its research, mostly private, and eugenics organizations proliferated in the first three decades of this century. In 1910, Charles B. Davenport opened the Eugenics Record Office in Cold Spring Harbor, New York, an adjunct to the Station for Experimental Evolution supported by the Carnegie Institution. The Eugenics Record Office served for nearly three decades as an important center for the study of human heredity, a national resource for local eugenics societies, and a site for training social workers and teachers in eugenics research and education. The Human Betterment Foundation in Pasadena, California, directed by Paul Popenoe and Edwin Gosney, was the leading center for eugenics on the West Coast. Their studies of the success of California's sterilization program influenced a new wave of sterilization laws in the 1920s and 1930s, including the one passed in Vermont in 1931. Both the Galton Laboratory in England and the Eugenics Record Office at Cold Spring Harbor compiled findings from their massive studies into catalogs of human heredity. International conferences provided an opportunity for exchange of ideas and the development of professional connections. Hundreds of colleges and universities in the United States and Europe introduced eugenics into their curricula in the areas of biology, social work, public health and medicine, and "sex hygiene." Eugenics societies enlisted the support of churches, patriotic organizations, private charities, and state welfare agencies to promote research and education in eugenics.[3]

While eugenicists did not always agree on research methods and interpretation of findings, the eugenics language and conceptual framework established a tradition in which most issues of the day, ranging from war to child welfare, were interpreted and debated in terms of human heredity and reproductive trends. Theodore Roosevelt, for example, attacked pacifist-eugenicist David Starr Jordan, president of Stanford University, who had argued that war was "dysgenic" because it removed the strongest men from the national breeding stock and left the draft rejects to father the next generation. Likewise, intellectuals debated women's rights, sexual freedom, social welfare programs, and race relations in eugenic or dysgenic terms (see fig. Intro. 1).[4]

A movement that encompassed so many disciplines and claimed authority for the direction of human evolution is bound to have its dissenters from within and without. Eugenics was never as unified as its leaders proclaimed. The 1930s represent a period of dissension and reform within the eugenics movement in Britain and the United States. Advances in genetics and medicine, criticism of eugenics research and propagandist campaigns, and a sensitivity to the race and class prejudices, heightened by Hitler's translation of eugenics into a national race hygiene program, all contributed to reforms within the movement. Proponents of the "new eugenics" of the 1930s stressed

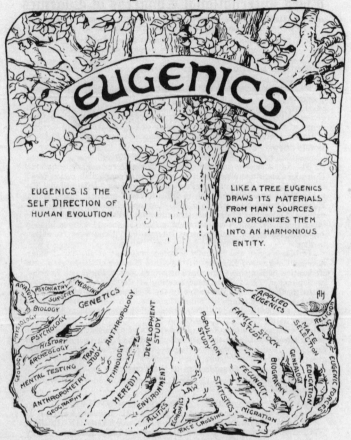

Eugenics Congress Announcement
Number 1. History and Purpose of the Congress.

EUGENICS

EUGENICS IS THE SELF DIRECTION OF HUMAN EVOLUTION.

LIKE A TREE EUGENICS DRAWS ITS MATERIALS FROM MANY SOURCES AND ORGANIZES THEM INTO AN HARMONIOUS ENTITY.

Third International Eugenics Congress
New York City, August 21-23, 1932.

Intro. 1 Harry Laughlin, Director of the Eugenic Record office, prepared this tree image in 1931. While it expressed the interdisciplinary nature of eugenics, the idea of unity was an illusion, concealing controversies over the interpretation of eugenics research and a growing disenchantment, among researchers in all relevant fields, with eugenic solutions to human problems. The Nazi adoption of eugenics as a program of race hygiene, and Laughlin's support for it, spelled doom for the unity of American eugenics and for Laughlin's own career. Announcement of the Third International Congress of Eugenics, New York City, 1932. Eugenics Survey of Vermont papers, Vermont Public Records Office.

the role of environment in shaping intellect and behavior, eliminated the rhetoric of racial inequality, condemned anti-Semitism, and abandoned analogies between animal breeding and human betterment. While some eugenicists adhered to the old, or "mainline," eugenics, the new eugenics enjoyed the support of scientists and maintained a notable constituency after World War II. The American Eugenics Society continued to revise its eugenic mission in response to scientific and political developments through the 1960s, as it supported research on world population problems, birthrates, and birth control; genetics counseling; and "social biology." Still, the "old eugenics" cast a long shadow on enterprises concerning the quality of the human gene pool, and the term was finally abandoned after 1970.

The Eugenics Survey of Vermont was part of this international movement. Henry F. Perkins, chairman of the University of Vermont (UVM) Zoology Department, organized the Eugenics Survey of Vermont in 1925 as an outgrowth of a heredity course. Under Perkins's direction, social workers hired by the privately funded survey conducted eugenic studies of Vermont families and communities over the next eleven years. Perkins publicized their findings in annual reports to support a broad range of social reforms in the state in the areas of child welfare, education, and charities and corrections. Most notorious of these reforms was Vermont's Sterilization Law of 1931. Perkins expanded the Eugenics Survey in 1928 into the Vermont Commission on Country Life, a comprehensive study of the social, cultural, and economic forces influencing the quality of family and community life in rural Vermont. The commission's final report, *Rural Vermont: A Program for the Future* (1931), became a working plan for rural rejuvenation and human betterment in Vermont communities. In the 1930s the Eugenics Survey focused on the "immigrant question." Sociologist Elin Anderson, assistant director of the Eugenics Survey and instructor of eugenics in the UVM Zoology Department, directed a four-year study of ethnic relations in Burlington. Published in 1937, Anderson's *We Americans: A Study of Cleavage in An American City* illustrates a dramatic transformation in the purpose and meaning of eugenics in Vermont.

The archive of the Eugenics Survey and the Vermont Commission on Country Life—over forty cartons of manuscripts, raw data, and source material generated by these organizations—was cataloged and preserved, through a grant Harry Perkins obtained from the Historical Records Division of the Works Progress Administration in 1936. The records were ultimately deposited in Vermont Public Records in 1952, where they remained, largely neglected until the past decade. Interest in the Eugenics Survey was aroused as Vermont historians and journalists examined the realities behind the myths of Vermont's past during bicentennial celebrations. The Eugenics Survey of Vermont and the Vermont Commission on Country Life emerged as a focal point for confronting the racism, xenophobia, and religious intolerance beneath the mythical portrayals of Vermonters as a "hardy race" descended from the old New England Protestant stocks. Inspired by the rising interest in the Holocaust, artists and journalists have adopted the Nazi metaphor and portrayed the Eugenics Survey as Vermont's counterpart to the Shoah. Perkins has since become a distillation of all the anxieties and pathologies of our time.[5]

Harry Perkins might have escaped this censure had he not worked so hard to define Vermont's people in eugenic terms and to turn his enterprise into a "program for the future" of the state, devoted to the conservation of Vermont's Yankee Protestant heritage. But the exclusion of some Vermonters from that future, through the Eugenics Survey's promotion of negative eugenics, lies beneath the veneer of Vermont's pastoral images and traditional country life, promoted by Vermont artists, authors, and the tourist board. Most poignant of all is the plight of the Abenaki Indians, the original inhabitants of Vermont. Many members of Abenaki families who were investigated by the Eugenics Survey were also incarcerated in institutions and subsequently sterilized. It was the Eugenics Survey, Abenaki leaders insist, that forced Abenaki families to conceal their identity, leave their ancestral homeland, or relinquish their language, religion, and customs. For Vermont Abenakis, eugenics was neither science nor a program of human betterment; it was an agent of their annihilation.[6]

Confronted with the multiplicity of interpretations of Harry Perkins and the Eugenics Survey, I sought first to understand the Eugenics Survey projects within their local, professional, and scientific contexts through constructing a detailed chronology of the investigations, the sources that informed them, and their products. This book is the result of that endeavor. Unlike some local studies of eugenics, this is not a history of sterilization in Vermont, nor is it an analysis of gender, race, and class prejudices, power relations, or the false science of the Eugenics Survey. This book seeks first to integrate the Eugenics Survey of Vermont into its forgotten context within Vermont's era of progressive reform. Second, it seeks to place the Eugenics Survey within the broader history of the eugenics movement. Harry Perkins rarely appears in histories of American eugenics, despite his leadership of the American Eugenics Society in 1931–1934. Elazar Barkan, in *The Retreat of Scientific Racism* (1992), noted that the transitional years (1929–1933) from the old, or mainline, eugenics to new, or reformed, eugenics form a "lacuna" in our historical understanding of eugenics and warrant further investigation.[7] This book will document that development as experienced in Vermont.

Chapter 1 examines the life and career of Eugenics Survey director Harry Perkins, whose intellectual history, family values, and cultural traditions established and shaped his work in eugenics. Chapter 2 traces Vermont economic, social, and political developments from 1890 to 1925, which provided the rationale and infrastructure for the survey. I will examine the emergence of eugenics thinking among progressive social reformers, social workers, and public officials during a period when the relations between state and local governments were being modernized. Chapter 3 examines the Eugenics Survey projects and publications from 1925 to 1931, as Harry Perkins struggled to adapt his eugenics enterprise to local concerns and changing attitudes in medicine, biology, and social work. Chapter 4 describes how Harry Perkins and his assistant, Elin Anderson, confronted the political turmoil and controversies over eugenics in the 1930s and documents the submergence of eugenics in social work, biology, and public welfare in the 1940s.

This study has a philosophical dimension as well. When a society finds its security, its prosperity, or its future quality of life threatened, causes are sought; studies are made; solutions based on those findings are offered. The boundary between private rights and the public interest is a negotiable one. How private and personal matters collected in confidence became transformed into problems of public urgency that justified radical intrusions on private life is one of the themes of this book. We find ourselves somewhere between a past we have condemned and a future in which we have invested tremendous resources in the collection of genetic data and its digestion in endless studies that define our humanity and predict our future health.[8] As eugenics sentiments emerge, as they frequently do, our best safeguard against the injustices of the past rests with our willingness to confront our connection to this history prior to disowning it and with our recognition of the enduring power of research findings and the consensus of experts over our perceptions of other people's problems.

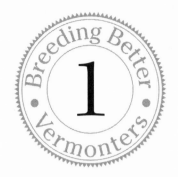

The Making of a Eugenicist: Henry F. Perkins, 1877–1925

The Land where we were born is wondrous fair,
    An Emerald Jewel in the iron crown
Of the rugged North, fit for a storied place
    Within the whole earth's royal treasury;
Won from the wilderness by our fathers' toil,
    Sealed ours by their blood and loyalty.

**—Helen M. Judd, "To the Daughters of Vermont
in Boston"**

The finest expression of national loyalty any man or woman can make is that which is manifested by devotion to the interests of his state in doing well the work nearest at hand . . . our State University will make Vermont vibrant with its lofty purposes and its splendid accomplishments; the nation will rejoice with us in our prosperity and the whole world will honor us for the product of an intelligent, efficient, and righteous manhood and womanhood.

—Guy Potter Benton, Inaugural Address, 1910

Without Henry F. Perkins, there probably would never have been a eugenics survey of Vermont. For it was Professor Perkins who discovered in eugenics the means to renew Vermont's heroic history and reveal the sources of Vermont's social and economic problems. The story of how Harry Perkins came to such a realization began at his birth in 1877 into a Protestant culture that saw itself as an expression of science and humanism, in a state whose history embodied the ideals and tradition of American democracy, and into a family that personified them all. Henry Perkins's career, when understood within the historical context of one of the most revolutionary periods in the history of science, reveals the inevitable tensions of a generation that struggled to understand the human implications of modern biology.

Born in 1877 and educated during the post-Darwinian controversies of the late nineteenth century, Perkins became a zoology professor at the dawn of the "Mendelian Revolution" and died in 1956, a few years after the molecular structure of DNA and the "central dogma" of James Watson and Francis Crick launched a new revolution in genetics. His shift from observations of birds and invertebrates to field studies of human populations was a logical one for the professional culture in which he lived and taught. His academic interest in eugenics rested on a well-cultivated belief that biology offered the best understanding of the human condition and the liberal Protestant belief that all knowledge should be directed toward improvement of the human condition in this life rather than toward seeking redemption in the next.

One of the most outstanding facts of Harry Perkins's life is that he lived nearly his entire life in the home where he grew up, two blocks from the University of Vermont campus green. His identity was firmly entrenched in family reputation, his elite neighborhood, the church and clubs that were integral to this insular world, and the University of Vermont (UVM), of which his home was an extension. All dimensions of Harry's life conspired to reinforce the traditions, values, and obligations of the Protestant Yankee elite culture and erected formidable boundaries to understanding or appreciating people who lived outside this world. When the twentieth century brought social and cultural changes that challenged the security, authority, and continuity of this way of life, eugenics offered one means of preserving it.

Three patterns dominate Harry Perkins's professional career and his public life. First, he was inclined to "color within the lines," a trait that served him well professionally and secured his position as a leader in good standing in the university community. Less likely to question authority (until scientific or public opinion demanded it) than to distinguish himself within the prevailing consensus, Harry Perkins periodically found himself in the wake of scientific advance instead of on its cutting edge. When scientific consensus shifted, as it did nearly every decade during his career, he experienced his most creative moments, as he found ways to repackage his teaching and research as though he had been on the leading edge of scientific progress all along.

Second, Perkins was proud. Prestige and reputation guided his professional and social connections, his choice of projects, and his service to the institutions that projected his identity. He rarely ventured beyond more distinguished circles professionally and socially to confide in personal matters, solicit advice, or socialize. Often inflating the importance of his projects, he became a bold and effective promoter and fund-raiser for projects he endorsed, a sort of impresario figure. His pride in the Eugenics Survey led him to preserve its archive in its entirety and extol its role in bringing about the most important Progressive reforms in the state. If pride was his Achilles heel, it could also be his salvation. His quest for respect forced him to abandon ideas that fell into disrepute along with his colleagues who held them.

Finally, a colleague posthumously referred to Harry Perkins as a "dilettante," a description that pleases his detractors immensely and has come to signify all his ventures, especially eugenics. His records support such a contention, for he took up a great many projects that he never saw through to completion, spread his efforts into diverse fields, and seemed to have only a superficial and unsophisticated understanding of them. He saw himself, however, as a visionary and a "pathfinder," whose purpose was to lead the way and let others work out the details of implementation. His dilettante style and broad scope of activities, however, concealed his deep and abiding commitment to a constellation of values and traditions, of which all his projects were manifestations.

Privileged Childhood in a State of Nature, 1877–1894

Henry Farnham Perkins was born in Burlington, Vermont, on May 10, 1877, the only son of George Henry Perkins and Mary Farnham Perkins. Members of prominent families who had founded the town of Galesburg, Illinois, the newly wedded couple had moved to Burlington in 1870 when George was hired as professor of natural history at UVM. As Congregationalists and highly educated descendants from the old New England stock, they shared with prominent Burlington families a distinguished ancestry of ministers, farmers, and entrepreneurs who were increasingly celebrated after the Civil War as the people who had built the republic. Harry's parents nurtured his appreciation of nature and cultivated his understanding of his place and purpose in life by instilling in him humanistic values, scientific vision, and missionary zeal—a combination that would reach full expression in his utopian dream of the Vermont Commission on Country Life.[1]

The Perkins family exemplified the late-nineteenth-century trend in the upper and middle classes toward smaller families, in which parents correspondingly invested a greater interest in the well-being and education of their children. Harry was an only child, his sister Harriet (1871–1876) having died from diphtheria a year before he was born. In his education, his opportunities in life, his residence in the finest neighborhood in Burlington, and the devotion of his parents, Harry was certainly blessed with an indulged youth. He grew up with all the privileges—and expectations—of the small, affluent family. Like many old New England families, Harry's ancestors had come to America in the seventeenth century and had taken advantage of the opportunities offered during the westward expansion. As "pioneer stocks" became scattered throughout the country, relatives were united by correspondence between siblings, cousins, aunts, and uncles, and family identity was defined by genealogies that traced family lineage to the colonial period and the American Revolution. Harry's "extended kinship network," bound by heredity and history to the accomplishments of their ancestors, translated into an obligation to continue the leadership and proprietorship of the American institutions they created. This rather heady history served to instill values of personal achievement, responsibility, and civic duty as indicators of human worth, with distinction in government, church, and academia as the manifestation of their development. At the same time, they frequently invoked the pioneering spirit of their ancestors, who symbolized initiative, tenacity, and vision.

To young Harry, his father, George Perkins, might have seemed the incarnation of the Founding Father. Having benefited from the growth of institutions of higher learning and a greater investment in science and professional knowledge, George Perkins became an important figure in the university and in the state. Private endowments and land grants from the Morrill Act gave him an endowed Chair of Natural Sciences and enabled him to enlarge the natural science program and create a museum of Vermont's geological, zoological, and archaeological treasures. Remembered as the father of the modern science curriculum at UVM, the elder Perkins was appreciated as well for his efforts to bring scientific knowledge to the service of the people. He gave public lectures, published articles on Vermont natural history, and served as state geologist and state entomologist. While creating for himself a place in the university history, he fashioned a niche for his son, to whom he gradually turned over his titles and responsibilities. Yet George never relinquished his paternal position. Until his death at age eighty-nine, Harry was the son in his father's house. He had been his father's Sunday school pupil and his father's science student in college. Harry became a zoology professor in the College of Arts and Sciences where his father served as dean, in the university where his father acted as vice president and interim president during World War I. While Harry was not as much admired or appreciated as his father, comparisons of the achievements of father and son recede into insignificance in the face of their strong filial devotion, their mutual commitment to their family, their church, and their professional reputations, and their efforts to expand the influence of all three throughout the state.[2]

In addition to expanding natural science education from the university into Vermont communities, George Perkins pioneered the teaching of Darwinian evolution at the University of Vermont. The challenge of the Civil War to the security and order of American life had been compounded by the publication of Darwin's *Origin of Species* (1859) and its implications for the moral and religious order of human life. The rupture of the symbiosis of science and religion, so secure in the Anglo-American Protestant tradition of natural theology, played out in the arena of the "post-Darwinian controversies" of the last four decades of the nineteenth century. George Perkins, like most Congregationalists, found a reconciliation in "Christian Darwinism." This interpretation of evolution assumed that natural selection was the instrument of God's creation, and the continuing force of natural selection in the present was evidence of God's ongoing immanence in both human and natural history. The human mind and "soul" became the material expression of selection forces modifying nerve tissue into an organ capable of reason, foresight, and imagination.[3]

For George Perkins, the pursuit of natural history from a Darwinian perspective was as much an expression of his religious faith and his Protestant commitment to human progress as it was a scientific endeavor. Teaching Sunday school at the College Street Congregational Church and teaching university students zoology, geology, and anthropology served in complementary ways to fulfill his Christian obligation.[4] Unlike the next generation, for whom Darwin's theories would become a source of anxiety and contentious debates, the Christian Darwinists of George Perkins's generation found the idea of human "creation" by means of natural selection self-validating. The theory confirmed biologically what was evident to them historically, that Christian "civilized" societies owed their dominance in the world to their adaptability and mental capacity for altruism and complex social organization. History, religion, and biology became fused in Christian Darwinism to replace the older Protestant assertion of their moral superiority with nature's confirmation of their more highly evolved intellectual capabilities and "social instincts." George Perkins used classic Christian Darwinian texts in his biology classes and apparently incorporated that perspective into his anthropology course.[5]

Harry Perkins's mother, Mary Farnham, exemplified the feminine complement of Yankee Protestant achievement. She graduated from Knox College in Galesburg, a private coeducational college that had been the site of a Lincoln-Douglas debate in 1858. In college she organized student seminars around such diverse topics as comparative religions and "embryology," for which she received a bachelor's degree in 1863. Her enthusiasm for academics carried over into church activities, where she became deeply inter-

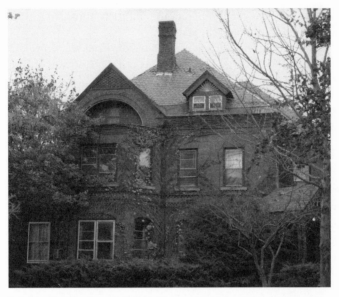

1.1 The Perkins house, 205 South Prospect Street, Burlington, Vermont.

ested in foreign missionary work. Mary Perkins brought the same dedication and leadership to church and civic service in Burlington. She became a deacon in the College Street Congregational Church and a director of the Vermont chapter of the Board of Missions of the Congregational Church. She served on the board of managers of the Home for Destitute Children for many years, until her death in 1904. A devoted mother and a supportive companion in her husband's travels and fieldwork, Mary Farnham was eulogized as possessing "the training of a pioneer. . . . She dressed well, she wrote well, she talked well, and tho attempting to spare others, she never spared herself in whatever the Church asked of her."[6] While George Perkins presented a model of triumph and proprietorship over nature and human institutions, Harry's mother represented the synthesis of nature and nurture—in home, family, and philanthropy. Harry absorbed his mother's interest in foreign missionary work and social programs for children. From her strength came his respect for women as intellectual equals, as competent scholars and social leaders, and as independent thinkers.

The large brick-and-stone house George Perkins designed and built on South Prospect Street in 1885 (see fig. 1.1) signified social station at the apex of the Burlington community. For Harry, it was home, the reflection of his birthright; the manifestation of the character, cultivation, and taste brought by civilization; and his entitlement to the respect and deference of others. As South Prospect Street and Burlington hill society presented Harry with a

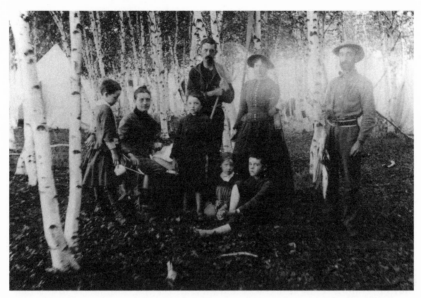

1.2 Young Harry absorbed his father's teaching of natural history and a love for Vermont's scenic retreats during family excursions into the "wilderness," such as this one in Swanton, Vermont, in the 1880s. Mary and George Perkins (*standing*) and young Harry (*sitting*) are the family on the right. George H. Perkins Papers, University of Vermont Archives. Courtesy Special Collections Department, University of Vermont Library.

model of civilization, Vermont's pristine woods, picturesque mountains and valleys, and rocky shores along Lake Champlain served as the venue for Harry's initiation into nature study and appreciation of Vermont's finest resources. Young Harry's excursions into Vermont's "wilderness" involved camping with his family while his father collected Indian bones and artifacts on archeological sites or surveyed geological formations (see fig. 1.2). Later, the family spent summers at Eagle Camp in the Lake Champlain islands, where summer programs in natural history were offered to Vermont students and teachers. Throughout life, Harry's appreciation for the places of memory in his childhood—"nice living" in town and unspoiled scenery in the country —became the defining themes in his photography, his research, and finally his interpretation of eugenics.[7]

Undergraduate Study: University of Vermont, Class of '98

For a son of George Perkins, the rite of passage into adulthood was a college degree, followed by a doctorate from a prestigious American university.

Harry's initiation began with a bachelor's degree in the classical curriculum, the most prestigious and scholarly course of study and the one that was believed to provide the best preparation for the future leaders of American democratic institutions. While the classical curriculum was the most intellectually broadening, it was also the most traditional. Within that program, Harry came to understand the purpose of his higher education, the importance of its traditions and values to modern progress, and his obligations as an adult. It was to that program that Harry would return in 1902 to build his own career and sustain and develop its underlying philosophy in his own teaching. And it was from that tradition that eugenics education and research emerged in Vermont.[8]

The classical curriculum at the University of Vermont rested on a philosophy established by UVM president James Marsh in the early nineteenth century, one that endured in principle until after World War II despite the periodic restructuring of departments and colleges into more specialized fields of study. The Marsh curriculum attempted to create balance and unity among the academic study of literature, classical languages, natural science, and philosophy. Coherence was achieved through a foundation in the classics, from which, presumably, all modern knowledge of nature, mankind, ethics, philosophy, and religion was ultimately derived. Philosophy stood at the apex of the university experience, when students' knowledge and maturity had been properly developed to reflect intelligently on the larger questions of human existence.[9]

By the 1890s the unity of the Marsh curriculum had begun to disintegrate in response to the modernizing trends towards specialization in all fields and the demand for a more pragmatic and technical education to serve the needs of scientific agriculture in a growing industrial, capitalist economy. Undergraduates in the classical curriculum were encouraged to select a field of concentration, yet advanced courses in history, philosophy, social and political science, and natural science retained an emphasis on the larger philosophical questions about man and nature that each subject inspired. During Harry's college years, the professors of the classical curriculum numbered only fourteen. They shared a long tenure and pride in developing the curriculum to preserve the integrity of the Marsh philosophy despite apparent modernization of the curriculum.

The progressive development of mankind from primitive to modern civilized societies provided the unifying theme of the classical curriculum in the 1890s. In sociology, Harry learned the theories of Comte and Spencer while his father's anthropology class surveyed the "ethnological, social, moral, and intellectual characteristics of the principal races of the world" and the "origin and development of modern social, religious, commercial, and political institutions."[10] Life sciences rested on the foundation of Professor Perkins's

Christian Darwinism. University president Buckham taught political economy and constitutional history, endowing his students with a Congregational minister's appreciation for the institutions for which they presumably would assume responsibility. Professors' homes were an extension of the Classical College, where students occasionally met for seminars or dined with their professors. This intimacy initiated students into the intellectual and social culture of traditional academe, shielded them from the more impersonal and technological influences of the modern age, and recognized their privileged position within the student body.[11]

While the classical curriculum cultivated Harry's intellectual commitment to the university traditions, the flowering of social life and campus rituals in the 1890s created a sense of loyalty to the institution and forged emotional bonds among students and alumni. Founder's Day observances, initiated in 1892, were held annually on Ira Allen's birthday or in conjunction with "Old Home Week" in Burlington. The ceremonies instilled in students an appreciation for the history and traditions of the university, by presenting their academic and social experience as the fulfillment of a century-old vision for Vermont.[12] Intercollegiate athletics, school colors and songs, and an expansion of fraternities and sororities were the contribution of Harry's generation to the twentieth century. Harry's graduating class inaugurated a tradition that would grow over the next six decades into the main campus event of the year. "Kulled Koon's Kake Walk" began as a minstrel show in which fraternities competed in a theatrical performance of what was billed as an old southern plantation ritual. Harry and a fraternity brother competed in the first of these annual events. (Abandoned in the wake of the 1960s civil rights movement, it left an indelible stamp of racism on the university history.)[13] Harry took an active part in many other areas of campus social life as well. Delta Psi fraternity, the debating club, the YMCA, and military drill (the forerunner of ROTC) provided a complement to the rigors of academe, while nurturing its traditional values through encouraging leadership and building character. Attendance at religious observances at UVM had become voluntary in the 1890s, but membership in the YMCA was encouraged to provide students with opportunities for Bible study, community service, and spiritual, physical, and social development. Harry remained an active member of the YMCA throughout his graduate years at Johns Hopkins, represented the organization at national conferences, and continued to nurture the UVM chapter as a young professor.[14]

Harry completed the first phase of his rite of passage with distinction. He graduated as a Phi Beta Kappa member in 1898 (see fig. 1.3) and was accepted into Johns Hopkins University's doctoral program in zoology to study under William Keith Brooks, the most distinguished American professor of zoology of the nineteenth century. Yet Harry's interest in biology was not so

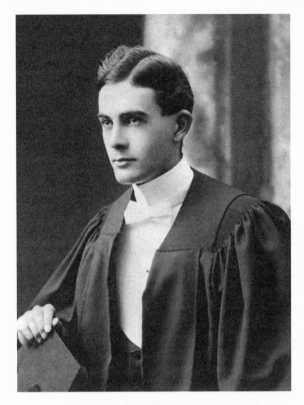

1.3 Henry F. Perkins, class of 1898, University of Vermont.
George H. Perkins Papers, University of Vermont Archives. Courtesy Special Collections Department, University of Vermont Library.

narrowly focused that he could not proudly display the interdisciplinary mission of the classical curriculum. His commencement address, "Education and the Labor Problem," indicates an early interest in the topics that would take center stage in the Progressive era, but his next serious encounter with such topics would be from the perspective of a zoology professor, with a particular interest in eugenics.

Biological Foundations at Johns Hopkins University, 1898–1902

Under the direction of Professor William Keith Brooks, Johns Hopkins's natural history program had become legendary. In the 1880s and 1890s, Brooks's program of graduate study received aspiring biologists from all over the United States and abroad. His students' dissertations were readily published and their credentials enabled them to secure academic positions in American universities and opportunities for research abroad. Brooks's impressive roster of students included Thomas Hunt Morgan, whose leadership at Columbia led to the development of the chromosome theory of heredity; Ross Harrison, E. B. Wilson, and E. G. Conklin, who led biologists into the era of experimental cytology and embryology; and William Bateson, who popularized Mendelian genetics in England. All attributed their success to Brooks's inspiration to study the "big questions" concerning the nature of heredity and its role in evolution.[15]

William Keith Brooks (1848–1908) was an embryologist and a committed Darwinian whose research and philosophy epitomized the late-nineteenth-century tradition of natural history, in which hypothetical evolutionary relationships were deduced from detailed comparisons of structure, embryonic development, and life cycles of plants and animals. Brooks had published major studies in marine biology and had developed the Chesapeake Zoological Laboratory in the 1880s into an active educational and research program stressing original research. In Brooks's marine zoology laboratory students learned to become careful, meticulous observers of organisms in their natural habitat. Original research consisted of collecting, observing, illustrating, and describing in detail a selected species' morphological development throughout its life cycle, with particular attention to its unique adaptations to the environment. From that data, the probable ancestral relationships and evolutionary history were deduced. Brooks demanded independence in his students, believing that scientific knowledge emerged within a struggle with particular questions and the resulting perception of patterns and relationships that emerge through observation. Harry Perkins's dissertation on the reproductive adaptations of a particular species of jellyfish displays the diligent observation, detailed illustrations, and conservative interpretations that characterize this tradition.[16]

As a naturalist, Brooks had no tolerance for laboratory experimentation as a means of understanding the nature of life phenomena. Life, he believed, revealed its mysteries through the reciprocal interaction of environmental influences and inherited variations, a phenomenon best understood through observations in the field, not through artificial manipulation of organisms or embryos in the laboratory. But it was in the laboratory and experimental breeding studies that some of these mysteries were revealing themselves to some of Brooks's own students, who attributed their success to a major departure from their mentor's ideas. Experiments on cells, embryos, and regeneration of body parts offered new approaches to understanding the mechanisms of heredity and development. In 1900, Mendel's laws surfaced in experimental plant breeding studies and began the "Mendelian revolution," which gave birth to the science of genetics. But from the late 1890s until his death, Brooks became increasingly alienated from these new experimental research programs. As it was, Harry Perkins had entered Johns Hopkins at the twilight of Brooks's distinguished career, when his reaction to the younger generation's abandonment of the field for the laboratory was to insulate his own students from these influences and dismiss them as dead ends in the quest for biological understanding.[17]

During Perkins's years at Johns Hopkins, Brooks was entering his "philosophical" period, when he was writing mostly on the nature of science, its epistemology, and its meaning for those engaged in the study of life. In 1899 he published *Foundations of Zoology*, which served as a point of departure for student research and Thursday evening discussions of philosophy and zoology at his home. *Foundations* was more a reflection on the *study* of nature than on its substance. Life, Brooks argued, is distinguished by the continual adjustment to environmental conditions. The biologist studies those responses and can understand them through his experience of living things in their natural environment. The history of life on earth is indeterminate, governed neither by necessity nor intrinsic causes. Scientific knowledge, then, is always tentative; "scientific laws" are simply observed regularities that are particularly useful to humans in their struggle for existence. Explanations of "ultimate reality" lie within the domain of metaphysics or theology rather than science. For Brooks, the study of evolutionary relationships in biology was a confrontation with the underlying unity of all life forms, including mankind. Brooks was not a pure materialist, yet he viewed human consciousness and intelligence as products of natural selection acting throughout human history. The human capacity for reason, the human awareness of individual "free will," and the human sense of "moral responsibility" were, in Brooks's view, adaptive responses.[18]

In the 1890s, Brooks had adopted one important contribution from experimental embryology, however, which placed Harry Perkins's graduate training within the turn-of-the-century tradition of "neo-Darwinism": August Weismann's theory of hard heredity. Because evolution theories depended on inherited variations, a theory of heredity that explained the phenomena of reproduction and development and the observed patterns in nature became an all-important goal of biologists. Lamarckian theories of soft heredity, which prevailed in the nineteenth century, proposed mechanisms by which parents' acquired habits, strengths or weaknesses, or damage from injury or disease became incorporated into the reproductive cells as they were manufactured. The offspring would presumably inherit the effects of their parents' efforts and experience. In the 1890s, German cytologist August Weismann introduced the concept of the "germplasm" to refute all such theories. Inspired by studies on the behavior of chromosomes in cell division and fertilization, Weismann proposed that the parents' bodies were simply the *vehicles* of the hereditary material, or the germplasm (consisting of particles on the chromosomes) produced independently from the other cells in the body (the somatoplasm) through cell division. The germplasm was immortal (as long as it was

propagated through reproduction) and was not altered by the parents' behavior or environment. Variations within a population resulted solely from
recombination of particles in the germplasm through sexual reproduction.
Neo-Darwinians used Weismann's theory to defend their belief that natural
selection, alone, directed evolution, against contenders (like Herbert Spencer
and the Mendelians) who proposed alternative mechanisms of heredity and
evolution.[19]

Weismann's germplasm theory had profound implications for human biological evolution and the idea of human progress, because one's biological potential became constrained by the immutable germplasm of one's ancestors,
which no amount of striving, healthy living, or education could change. In the
neo-Darwinian view, human biological (racial) progress would depend entirely on self-imposed reproductive selection. It is no accident that Francis
Galton invented eugenics from a commitment to his own theory of hard
heredity. What the germplasm consisted of, how it operated in growth and
development, and how it created observed variations in natural populations
were matters of speculation in the 1890s, and most scientists remained un-
convinced of the central importance of either the germplasm or natural selection in development and evolution. But neo-Darwinians championed the
theory as the most important discovery since Darwin's. Brooks, in particular,
kindled his students' interest in the mysteries of heredity and encouraged
them to consider the broader philosophical implications of their studies.
"Many learned under him for the first time to take a philosophical look on zoological phenomena," reported George Lefevre, a student of Brooks from
1888 to 1898. "Most delightful of all is the recollection of long evenings on
the verandah, where, after the day's work was done, we sometimes sat listen-
ing to his talk on nature and philosophy."[20]

Harry Perkins completed his dissertation on the reproductive adaptations
of the jellyfish *Gonionema murbochii* in 1902 and, as was customary for
Brooks's students, published his findings that year. Upon graduation he was
offered the position of instructor of zoology at UVM. The privilege of being
the son of Professor George Perkins, then dean of Natural Sciences, had its
benefits as well as certain expectations. Dean Perkins, approaching sixty, was
eager to turn over a portion of his courses to his son and give Harry the ultimate gift of father to son: an opportunity that many a young Ph.D. at that
time would have considered a plum position.

In retrospect, this young professor launched his career with relatively little
exposure to and certainly no serious training in the research methods or theories that would ultimately define twentieth-century zoology. During the first
several years of Harry Perkins's career, however, these new developments
were still largely "works in progress," the subject of bitter controversies
among biologists and the basis for a variety of competing theories of heredity

and evolution.[21] The rewards for scientific originality and "revolt" from late-nineteenth-century natural history were not to be reaped until Harry Perkins had thoroughly settled into his niche as professor of zoology at UVM, where abandonment of academic tradition was hardly looked upon with great favor. During the first half of his teaching career, then, Dr. Perkins faced two challenges. He was given the zoology curriculum to develop at UVM and in so doing secure his position within the faculty. At the same time, Perkins had to educate himself in fields that had not been part of his graduate training and restructure his teaching and research accordingly. In both initiatives he proceeded conservatively, cautiously, and within the boundaries of biological consensus as presented in college textbooks and the established scientific journals and by recognized leaders in his field.

"Coming Home" to Vermont, 1902–1911

Upon returning home to the old neighborhood and to his alma mater, young Dr. Harry Perkins would find that little had changed. The aging President Buckham, a fixture since before Harry was born, continued to lead the faculty with the same collegial and paternalistic style, delivering his "sermons" on the virtues of humanistic education at university ceremonies and keeping records and correspondence with his famous quill pen. The professors of Harry's undergraduate days, the "classical" curriculum, the buildings, and the campus green remained as he had left them a few years before. The social organizations and campus rituals inaugurated in the 1890s were turning into more clearly defined, elaborate traditions. The university culture, its principles, and its historical connection with its founders endured despite major changes in the purpose and structure of higher education at work elsewhere. Harry returned from Johns Hopkins in 1902 not only with his doctorate but also with a fiancée. The following year he married Mary Edmunds, sister of one of his fellow graduate students and daughter of a prominent Baltimore family. They began their married life in a house on the same block where Harry was born. When Harry's mother died unexpectedly from pneumonia the following year, they moved into Dean Perkins's South Prospect Street house, where they made their permanent home.

The first ten years of young Dr. Perkins's career were productive and fulfilling. While teaching was his first and most important responsibility, he also engaged in research during the summer months. As a research assistant for the Marine Laboratory of the Carnegie Institution at Dry Tortugas, Florida (1902–1906), he maintained his connection with Brooks and other associates from Johns Hopkins. For Perkins, the seaside adventures were part of the naturalist's lifestyle and enriched his teaching more than his record of scholarly publication.[22] Family, campus and community life, and teaching occupied his time and interest more than research and scholarship. Yet as early as 1903 he was at least creating the appearance that his department was a research station with the letterhead he used in his professional correspondence. In Gothic letters it read: "Zoological Laboratory, University of Vermont, Burlington, Vermont."[23] In fact the "Zoological Laboratory" was more specifically an instructional laboratory for students than it was the research station the name implied. Yet for teaching purposes the lab made an important contribution. Nearly every course he developed emphasized laboratory work or field study, and he encouraged university support for students wishing to take advantage of summer opportunities for research at Wood's Hole, Massachusetts, and Cold Spring Harbor.

From 1902 until 1913, Dr. Perkins *was* the zoology department, and he continued to teach and serve as chairman as new faculty were added in ensuing years. Perkins developed the zoology curriculum on the Brooks model to the extent that he was able, while attempting to meet the needs of students in agriculture and premedicine. He expanded and diversified the course offerings in zoology; provided opportunities for original, independent study; and included an elective in scientific photography, enabling him to share one of his greatest passions with his students. By 1907 his teaching load had expanded to eight courses, which he taught without assistance until 1913. His promotions to assistant professor in 1906 and professor in 1911 coincided with the births of his two daughters.[24] (See fig. 1.4.)

Perkins's library acquisition records, his course descriptions, and the textbooks listed for those courses, suggest that he built the zoology curriculum on the Anglo-American naturalist tradition of Thomas H. Huxley and his followers, who attempted to establish a unified "science of life" set on a neo-Darwinian foundation. They offered a reconciliation of the historic tensions between natural history and physiology (medicine) and between laboratory and field research to demonstrate that all life phenomena, including human life, were explicable in terms of fundamental laws of nature. Perkins largely ignored experimental approaches in biology, except as filtered through their ambiguous and often skeptical presentation in these traditional biology texts. Classic works of the period on Mendelian genetics, new theories of animal behavior, and chemicals controlling growth and metabolism (named "hormones" in 1905) do not surface in his library records until 1912, nor do such topics appear in his course descriptions. While the vast majority of his library acquisitions consist of general and specific works in descriptive zoology and embryology, his records show a particular interest in evolution theory and its implications for human self-understanding. Perkins repeatedly borrowed such classics as Henry Fairfield Osborn's *From the Greeks to Darwin* (1899), G. J. Romanes's *Darwin and after Darwin* (1897), T. H. Huxley's *On the Ori-*

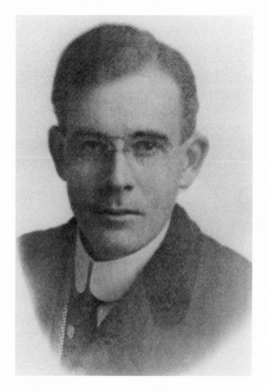

1.4 Harry Perkins as a young
professor. George H. Perkins Papers,
University of Vermont Archives.
Courtesy Special Collections Department, University of Vermont Library.

gin of Species (1883), Sir J. Arthur Thomson's *The Science of Life* (1899), and
Ernst Haeckel's *Last Words on Evolution* (1905). Defenses of Darwin's theory of natural selection and assertions of its significance to human history and
scientific progress, these works were treatises on the history, interpretation,
and philosophical importance of evolution theory, not rigorous analyses of
new research. Perkins's attraction to such works indicate his decision to teach
biology within the humanistic tradition of the Marsh curriculum.[25]

   *The Science of Life: An Outline of the History of Biology and Its Recent
Advances* (1899) by Sir J. Arthur Thomson of the Edinburgh School of Medicine's Zoological Laboratory, for example, was one staple in Perkins's library
record. A self-proclaimed neo-Darwinian, Thomson promoted a "modern biological attitude," which integrated the research in physiology, cell biology,
and embryology into the familiar framework of the naturalist and offered the
resulting synthesis as proof of Darwin's theory of evolution. Thomson emphasized the importance of field study, the interaction of organisms within
their environment, and the unity of all life revealed in the intricate relations
between structure and function at all levels of organization—from the chem-

istry of the protoplasm to human races and species. *The Science of Life* explained away the scientific controversies of the period as a vital sign of the healthy progress of biology as it had grown "from an embryonic state of relative insignificance to a central position among the sciences." Darwin's theory became the culmination of centuries of inquiry into the origin and nature of life. After a somewhat confused survey of competing theories of heredity, Thomson predicted that their resolution would reveal the final mystery of life: "The single statement which embraces the whole field of heredity must prove almost as epoch-making as the law of gravitation to the astronomer."[26]

Perkins also regularly borrowed Ernst Haeckel's *Last Words on Evolution*, a work whose purpose and content reveal a proto-eugenic orientation and suggest Perkins's intellectual solution to the religious implications of his neo-Darwinian worldview. Darwin's strongest advocate in Germany, Haeckel had fought religious opposition to evolution theory throughout his career. *Last Words* was a lecture he delivered in Berlin in 1905, provoked by the alleged "corruption" of Darwin's theory by Jesuit scholars who introduced the immortal soul into their teachings of evolution.[27] Haeckel claimed that the concept of a personal, immortal soul was an attempt on the part of men to fashion God in their own idealized image for political ends. "Soul" or "consciousness" was the product of a neurophysiology, which had an origin (conception), a chemical constitution (inherited in the germplasm of egg and sperm), and a material development. Mental incapacity or mental disease, Haeckel argued, were consequences of brain injury or abnormal development. In Darwinian fashion, Haeckel concluded that "the human soul, being material and physiological in nature, is subject to scientific investigation and has only reached its present height by a long period of evolution; it differs in degree, not in kind, from the soul of higher animals; and thus it cannot in any case be immortal." Religious teaching and beliefs, Haeckel asserted, "while ceasing to inform pure science," functioned as socializing and cultural forces, "the repertoire for art, poetry, and ethical inspiration and a sense of moral purpose." "Enlightened Protestants," he contended, had broadened the meaning of Christianity when they understood Jesus as a historical figure and discovered how religious teaching harmonized with "the splendid light of science."[28]

Perkins apparently cultivated that harmony himself, for he juxtaposed his reading and teaching of evolution with Bible study. Nearly every month he borrowed volumes of the *Cambridge Bible for Schools and Colleges*, an "enlightened Protestant" version with historical introductions and copious annotations, or *The Modern Readers' Bible*, which was edited to emphasize the literary qualities obscured in older translations. For Perkins, study of religion and biology had become complementary expressions of intellectual transcendence within a humanistic tradition.

Confronting Modern Change, 1910–1917

The University of Vermont entered a new era with the death of President Buckham in 1910. The hiring of his successor, Guy Potter Benton, acknowledged a desire on the part of the trustees to bring the university into the twentieth century. Benton's inaugural was celebrated with an unprecedented display of ceremony and was recognized by Vermont leaders as a historic "departure from the old order" and a commitment to modern progress in Vermont higher education.[29] In his inaugural address, Benton charted a new course for UVM, beginning with the modern need to abandon parochial sentimentality and "dethrone" the ultraconservativism and smug complacency of New England university culture. "State lines are only imaginary," Benton declared, "and the State is useful in largest measure only as it makes itself, with its own peculiar environment, of service to the people of the entire nation. There is no greater obstacle to individual and general progress than the curse of the local mind." Recognizing the sensitivities of the Vermont minority in his audience, Benton praised the unrivaled beauty of the state and the impressive character, history, and achievements of its people.[30]

Benton challenged the UVM faculty to refashion itself as a leader in modern university education and thereby renew Vermont's exalted position within the nation. Reverence for tradition, reliance on family connection and personal reputation, and the image "of scholars shut up in cloister or classroom," Benton promised, would be replaced with businesslike efficiency and cooperation with Vermont communities, state government, and industries. The university would initiate these partnerships, engage in public outreach, and offer its professional expertise to the state and to local communities. Benton charged each department with a specific role in the new mission. The social sciences, for example, should "study the relationship of pauperism to crime" and should project their educational programs "out into the crowded districts of the city and into the waste places of the country [and] make students, along with their teachers . . . active factors in improving the living conditions of all classes of people." Benton urged the College of Medicine to expand its horizons beyond diagnosis and treatment of diseases to the training of public health officials "who, in co-operation with the civil authorities of the community in which they may live and practice, shall become prominent factors in the prevention of disease." In scientific agriculture, Benton promoted the University of Wisconsin as the outstanding model among land grant colleges, the one UVM should emulate. For the College of Arts and Sciences, whose traditional role was to educate the future leaders of America, Benton assigned the somewhat vestigial function of cultivating "disciplined and appreciative minds."[31]

President Benton alienated the old guard at UVM while forcing them to confront the consequences of their ultra-conservatism. He substituted the corporate model of administration for Buckham's paternalistic one. Benton demoted the Department of Arts and Sciences by converting all the departments to colleges in 1911 and enlarging the funding, staff, and instructional program of the College of Agriculture. He supported the disturbing findings of the Carnegie Foundation's survey of education in Vermont (1912–1913), which had found the state system, at all levels "in want of adaptation" and unresponsive to the modern, practical needs of Vermont youth. The Carnegie fact finders criticized UVM for its failure to fulfill the "true spirit, meaning, and intent" of the Morrill Act, most notably in their diversion of state funds to support the arts and sciences at the expense of agriculture. Benton secured additional state funding for the establishment of regional agricultural extension stations "so that by cooperation between the trained specialists in the Agricultural College and the earnest farmers of the State we may make the barren and waste places of the state to blossom as the rose."[32]

These internal assaults on Perkins's traditional zoology curriculum coincided with scientific advances that challenged it from without. Harry's mentor, William Keith Brooks, who died in 1908, was lovingly celebrated in 1910 in the *Journal of Experimental Zoology* as a great teacher whose philosophy and methods of the study of life had come to an end. A new consensus embracing experimental zoology and Mendelian genetics was rapidly gaining momentum, with excitement over the discoveries of Thomas Hunt Morgan and his colleagues at the Columbia University "Fly Room." Drosophila studies confirmed the hypothesis that chromosomes were the material vehicles of "genes"; they were visibly altered in mutant forms and behaved predictably in accordance with Mendel's laws.[33] After 1912, "experimental" approaches in both basic and applied research dominated American biology. American biologists, having more readily adopted Mendelian genetics than their British counterparts, were receiving substantial support for genetics research from the Carnegie Institution and the American Breeders' Association. American geneticists conducted their research within two related but relatively autonomous fields: (1) basic research on experimental organisms, such as fruit flies, to understand how genes worked and (2) applied research in heredity to generate knowledge of the genetic basis of specific plant, animal, and human traits as revealed in breeding studies and pedigree analyses. Charles B. Davenport's Station for the Study of Experimental Evolution at Cold Spring Harbor and zoology departments at leading American universities—Harvard, University of Wisconsin, Stanford, University of California—were becoming centers for applied genetics and eugenics. With the proliferation of genetics and eugenics research, colleges and universities across the country began to integrate eugenics into biology, social work, psychology, and medical education. The naturalist tradition was not dead; it was simply fading into irrelevance as the experimental laboratory was yielding more interesting and useful information in the search for the mechanism of inheritance.

In 1913 the American Breeders' Association had changed its name to the American Genetics Association and instituted the *Journal of Heredity*, a serial on "Plant and Animal Breeding and Eugenics." Paul Popenoe, a Stanford-trained naturalist and an emerging leader in American eugenics, served as its first editor. While the *Journal of Heredity* was aimed at a general academic audience, in contrast to more technical biological publications, prominent biologists were well represented on its editorial board, a tradition that continued throughout its history. Zoologists and medical researchers became intimately involved in eugenics after 1910 and liberally contributed their expertise to social commentary and deliberations on public policy. Nearly all the familiar authors of Perkins's textbooks promoted eugenics, eventually serving as officers and advisors of eugenics organizations or authors of books and articles on this new "human biology."[34]

One such prominent biologist was David Starr Jordan, whose textbooks Perkins had used since 1902. Jordan, president of Stanford University, chaired the Eugenics Section of the American Genetics Association and in 1912 constituted a Committee to Study and to Report on the Best Practical Means of Cutting off the Defective Germ Plasm in the American Population. Its findings, based on a survey of physicians and a review of eugenics research, were presented in the Van Wagenen report of 1913. This report concluded that the American population was in fact deteriorating due to the proliferation of the feebleminded. The committee reported a general consensus of medical, biological, and legal opinion that sterilization of "defectives" was the most economical and humane solution to the apparent deterioration of the American population. After 1912 "applied research" in human heredity by leading American biologists became intimately connected to politics. Between 1907 and 1918 the first wave of eugenic sterilization laws were introduced into state legislatures, passed, and nearly all struck down.[35]

Harry Perkins must have understood the importance of Benton's demands for practical education and the new directions in American biology for his own teaching. Between 1911 and 1913, Perkins's library record shows an unprecedented surge of interest in works dealing specifically with heredity, evolution, and, for the first time, scientific works on genetics. He borrowed William E. Castle's and Charles B. Davenport's animal breeding studies, possibly in response to President Benton's initiatives to upgrade scientific agricultural education. Davenport's *Heredity in Relation to Eugenics* (1911) introduced Perkins to the work being done at the newly formed Eugenics Record Office at the Station for Experimental Evolution at Cold Spring Harbor.[36] Yet Perkins seemed unimpressed by breeding studies or the growing corpus of scientific literature from "experimental" research in zoology, for he showed a preference for the more familiar neo-Darwinian classics. He became most absorbed in the works of British zoologists Sir J. Walter Thomson and Sir Patrick Geddes and borrowed nearly every major work they had written.[37]

Thomson's *Heredity* (1908) presented eugenics within a framework that a disciple of W. K. Brooks and a zoology professor in the classical curriculum could appreciate. In *Heredity*, Thomson distinguished between environmentally induced "modifications" and inherited "variations," which, he argued, *interacted* to stimulate development and the expression of individual characteristics. Mankind, Thomson argued, being "slowly and slightly 'variable' is exceedingly 'modifiable'" and is "likely to have his inborn nature concealed by a veneer of nurture." Yet as humans were subject to the same laws as all life forms, Thomson noted, "we naturally look to Biology for some practical guidelines in relation to human affairs."[38]

Thomson urged physicians, sociologists, and biologists to collaborate to understand how environment and germplasm *interacted* to reveal particular genetic "predispositions" to health and disease (both mental and physical). While alleged "race poisons"—alcohol, opium, tobacco, the toxins of the microbe causing syphilis, or lead—might permanently damage the germplasm and cause truly inherited defects, Thomson rejected Lamarckian explanations. Such poisons, he argued, *modified* normal development in utero if they crossed the placental barrier or infected the mother during insemination. In that manner alcoholism, venereal disease, and other *environmental* factors were responsible for the high incidence of feebleminded, epileptic, alcoholic, or criminally insane offspring of parents who abused drugs or alcohol or had licentious lifestyles.[39] Criticizing Herbert Spencer's failure to distinguish between social and biological forces of "selection," Thomson urged biologists not to overlook the effects of social ostracism and bad working conditions in encouraging crime and alcohol abuse when considering genetic predispositions. Criminals, he ventured, might be simply "anachronisms," who found themselves outside their "optimal environment."[40] Low resistance to certain environmentally induced diseases, such as tuberculosis or gout, was probably inherited but could be prevented by proper sanitation, nutrition, and living conditions. "Racial health," in Thomson's view, required education, the "awakening of a eugenic consciousness" in the citizens, campaigns for improvement of housing, and a national program of public health.[41]

A program of eugenics, Thomson warned, must be conservative, "gentle,"and enlightened. It must seek to improve living conditions, both as an affirmation of human altruism and as a precondition to enable individuals from every rank of society to express the full range of their genetic potential. Thomson's interactionist paradigm did not, however, rule out future possibilities of a national program of eugenics. Genetic predispositions still were biological limitations, he emphasized through the words of William Bateson: "The stick will not make the dwarf peas climb, though without it the tall can never rise. Education, sanitation, and the rest are but the giving and withholding of opportunity."[42] But negative eugenics, in the form of segregation in institutions or marriage restriction, should apply only to those individuals who are "obviously unfit"—the idiot, the epileptic, the syphilitic, the lunatic —and those "who are totally dependent on public support." While Thomson conceded that such persons should "forfeit their right to reproduce," he protested "the impetuous recommendations of 'social surgeons' . . . who do not hesitate to recommend methods of surgical elimination to an extent that is almost grotesque."[43]

For Harry Perkins, Thomson's writings placed eugenics within a familiar, humanistic context and sustained the intellectual bias of the classical curriculum. More important, Thomson offered an interpretation of eugenics that preserved the key element of Perkins's training with Brooks and his teaching of evolution and embryology: the reciprocal influences of inherited variations and environment in the development of an organism. Perkins's own interests in child development would become an underlying theme in his eugenics research and education. While Thomson's *Heredity* has been invoked by some historians as a criticism of the overemphasis on heredity by "mainline" eugenicists, the available evidence strongly suggests that Thomson's interpretation helped to enlist the support of naturalist-oriented biologists such as Perkins for the so-called mainliner position, after a new consensus emerged over the truth of Mendelian genetics and an explosion of studies demonstrated the means to discover "genetic predispositions" to mental incompetence.[44]

In 1912, however, Perkins's response to the modern scientific challenge was to adopt the format of Thomson and Geddes. That year he introduced a new course: "Principles of Animal Biology," a one-hour elective featuring "Lectures and Reports" in "Properties of Living Substance, The Cell, Historical Study, Evolution."[45] Perkins changed its title to "Principles of Zoology" in 1914 and added "inheritance" to the topics listed in the course description. "Historical Study" became "History of Biology and Its Makers," after he read the book by William A. Locy with that title.[46] Limited to upperclassmen who had taken a previous course in zoology, "Principles" preserved the tradition of philosophical speculation on new knowledge. The "historical study" preserved the humanistic bias of the classical curriculum, offered a progressive view of modern biology, and provided the desired interdisciplinary coherence. For the liberal arts student, "Principles" provided the biological complement to advanced courses in sociology, psychology, philosophy, and anthropology, all of which featured the progressive development of civilization from savagery. More a course in science appreciation than in scientific training, "Principles" was Perkins's concession to modernization and his tribute to the ghosts of the founding fathers, from Marsh to Buckham.

While Perkins remained on the sidelines of the Mendelian revolution prior to World War I, he was not idle. He devoted considerable time and energy to raising a family, campus and community activities, and professional projects directed toward public service. He presided over the Bird and Botany Club and helped to organize the Boy Scouts, serving on its National Council and as chairman of the local council. He pursued his interest in color photography, invented a new development process for the Lumiere Company, and prepared exhibitions of his scenic photographs from his trips to Yellowstone and the Canadian Rockies. The Canadian Pacific Railroad hired Perkins to photograph the Canadian Rockies for their promotional literature and provided him with a private train for his laboratory. He served as UVM Phi Beta Kappa register, organized university ceremonies, and secured campus speakers. His scientific research consisted of a study sponsored by the State Fish and Game Commission on the effects of commercial fishing of lake shad on pike and other populations of "game fish" in Lake Champlain.[47] While these activities may seem incidental to his career as a eugenicist, or perhaps "dilettantish" for a scientist, they qualified as an appropriate fulfillment of a UVM professor's public service obligation. Such activities expanded his visibility and cultivated his interest in community affairs. Between 1912 and 1916, family and community appear to have taken precedence over academic research.

In 1916, Perkins took a sabbatical. Awarded the position of Fellow by Courtesy at Johns Hopkins University, he perhaps hoped to rekindle his enthusiasm for research. He once again took up, for the last time, his research on jellyfish. This endeavor proved instead to be the final chapter in his sporadic forays into marine biology. By this time, the eclipse of the naturalist tradition was nearly total. There is no evidence that Perkins ever published the results of his sabbatical work, nor did he leave any documentation of his year at Johns Hopkins. Perhaps during that year he became aware of the obsolescence of his earlier research and the scientific backwater his department had become.[48]

Upon his return to Burlington, Perkins resumed his regular teaching duties with no evident changes in his curriculum for two years. The war and the influenza epidemic occupied everyone's attention. Harry served in civilian defense during the war; his father became interim president while Benton served overseas in the American war effort. After the war, Dean Perkins's long and distinguished career was formally recognized by a fiftieth-anniversary celebration in recognition of his service to the university and to the state. The outpouring of tributes to his father may have inspired Harry to assume a more active and visible role in community and state affairs.[49]

While George and Henry Perkins attended to the war effort in their hometown, eugenicists and psychologists had launched a cooperative venture of their own. As men registered for military service and conscripts were processed at draft boards across America, new data were being collected. The particular "defects" of men rejected for service were recorded and registered in Washington, D.C. For the first time in U.S. military history, nearly two million recruits were given mental tests, purportedly to assist officers in determining duty assignments. The army Alpha and Beta mental tests were designed by a team of eugenicist-psychologists, led by Vineland Training School superintendent Henry H. Goddard, Harvard University psychology professor Robert M. Yerkes, and Stanford psychologist Lewis M. Terman, the architect of the 1916 Stanford-Binet test that measured IQ. This mass of new data in the years following the war would become fertile territory for eugenicists, who would analyze the distribution and relative incidence of particular "defects" and levels of "intelligence" according to region and state, race and nationality, and social class and background. It would also offer Harry Perkins an incentive to conduct eugenics research in Vermont.[50]

Professor Perkins's Emergence as a Eugenicist, 1921–1925

In 1919, Perkins restructured his zoology curriculum. He revised his "Principles of Zoology," a one-hour lecture course for juniors and seniors, with an updated content: "the cell, organs, systems of the animal body; embryology, heredity, instincts."[51] In 1921, "Principles of Zoology" became "Heredity: Lectures on the fundamental principles of zoology, the evolution of animals, genetics." "Heredity" was cross-listed in the School of Agriculture the following year, with a more practical emphasis: "Lecture course with conference and report exercises covering the principles of elementary embryology, the physical basis of inheritance, principles of breeding experiments, and eugenics, the practical application of heredity to mankind."[52] Although Perkins did not feature human genetics and eugenics in the Arts and Sciences course description until 1923, he taught these topics. The text Perkins used was Horatio H. Newman's *Readings in Evolution, Genetics, and Eugenics*. Newman's approach would guide Perkins's instruction and inspire his students' field investigations. Perkins was especially intrigued by Newman's studies of identical twins, which explored the relative influence of heredity and environment on development. Many of Perkins's students found the assignment to compare the life histories, physical features, and personalities of identical twins especially intriguing as proof of the genetic basis of human nature. Twin studies became the topic for at least one senior thesis and a master's thesis.[53]

While some historians have argued that eugenics began to wane in the 1920s, in college biology courses this was not the case. Eugenics was increasingly featured in zoology curricula at leading American universities in the 1920s. Harvard, Berkeley, the University of Wisconsin, Columbia, most of the Ivy League and midwestern and eastern state institutions taught eugenics in their zoology departments. Leading American geneticists wrote the textbooks, published frequently on eugenics, and presented papers at professional meetings. In addition to H. H. Newman's texts, Harvard geneticist William E. Castle's *Genetics and Eugenics* went through several editions between 1916 and 1930, as did University of Wisconsin geneticist Michael F. Guyer's *Being Well Born: An Introduction to Heredity and Eugenics*. Paul Popenoe and Roswell H. Johnson combined their professional expertise in biology and the social sciences in *Applied Eugenics*, whose first edition appeared in 1918. The new knowledge in genetics, chromosome theory, and experimental evolution, rather than undermining the tenuous claims of eugenicists that human evolution could be directed, served instead to give a broader, more "scientifically rigorous" base of support for such claims.

Perkins's choice of Newman's *Readings in Evolution, Genetics, and Eugenics* was a logical one, for it preserved the continuity of the neo-Darwinian tradition he had taught and rested on source material that Perkins had used in his courses during the first part of his teaching career. The first half of Newman's sourcebook is devoted to evolution theory, presented as a historical development of man's search for understanding the nature of life and as a demonstration of the growth and progress of biological thought from Darwin to "the modern attitude as to the truth of evolution doctrine." Newman had selected sources that demonstrated the compatibility of evolution and religion, recognizing "that even in these scientific days, the subject of evolution has a bad name in many communities and in educational institutions with religious affiliations."[54] Newman's "Genetics" section, roughly 30 percent of the text, surveyed all the research in heredity since 1900 and set the new discoveries within a historical development and conceptual framework that persist in most biology curricula today. Genetics was offered as the answer to the sixty-year search for a mechanism of heredity that explained the inherited sources of variability, the raw material for organic evolution. The "Evolution" and "Genetics" sections provided a powerful base of research and theory for the last and smallest section, "Eugenics," which consisted of only four chapters (sixty pages), roughly 12 percent of the course.

Human heredity, as presented in eugenics units in 1920s college textbooks, was an exercise in claiming "truth by empirical convergence." The "truth" of biological explanations for human diversity, health and disease, and the complexities of human nature rested, in these texts, on a powerful edifice of accumulated research in medicine, sociology, and biology. When a student had gained a firm grounding in cell theory, evolution, and plant and animal genetics, genetic explanations for specific human traits must have appeared logical. Twin studies, pedigree analyses, and statistical correlations conspired to substantiate genetic explanations for mental and social "defects." Eugenics, however, concerned the application of such knowledge to improving the national "racial" or "hereditary" health. Eugenics studies also demonstrated the social, economic, and public health problems resulting from propagation, through reproduction, of "diseased germplasm." Studies of such "hereditary defects" as feeblemindedness, epilepsy, and mental illness in particular families and ethnic groups or among the dependent or delinquent population suggested to the student particular technologies for reducing their incidence through reproductive control and immigration restriction.

No "mental defect" played a more crucial role in eugenics history than the condition known as "congenital feeblemindedness." In 1914, Henry H. Goddard, superintendent of the Vineland Training School for the Feebleminded in New Jersey, advanced a Mendelian explanation for the condition, which he published in his influential *Feeblemindedness: Its Causes and Consequences*. By 1916 his theory had found its way into the human heredity sections of biology textbooks.[55] Most clinical and legal definitions of feeblemindedness were some variation on that of the Royal College of Physicians (London): "One who is capable of earning his living under favorable circumstances, but is incapable from birth or from an early age of (a) competing on equal terms with his normal fellows or (b) of managing himself and his affairs with normal prudence."[56] In 1908, Goddard had traveled to Europe to study the causes and treatments of feeblemindedness and returned with French psychologist Alfred Binet's methods of measuring mental development, William Bateson's enthusiasm for Mendelian genetics, and the inspiration to turn his Vineland School into a research laboratory like the Galton Laboratory for National Eugenics.[57]

While Goddard had recognized the multiple causes of feeblemindedness, he nevertheless advanced a Mendelian explanation for the "life incompetence" of many of his charges, who seemed to have inherited their condition. Goddard hypothesized that mental retardation resulted from a single gene, which either prevented the production of a necessary substance for normal brain development or caused the production or accumulation of some inhibiting chemical. In subsequent studies, Goddard and others debated whether the gene was dominant, recessive, sex-linked, or influenced by other genes or environmental factors. Its relevant feature, however, was its traceability through family pedigrees, its roots in brain function, and its ability to attribute just about any behavior that was deemed "abnormal" to "subnormal" intelligence.

According to Goddard, "We know what feeblemindedness is, and we have come to suspect all persons who are incapable of adapting themselves to their environment and living up to the conventions of society or acting sensibly of being feebleminded."[58] Goddard's theory of feeblemindedness added the key element of biodeterminism that served to distill and explain in a unified way the diverse range of "symptoms" collected in the dockets of social workers. As the hypothetical "F" gene was traced through family histories, it offered a general explanation for any evidence of failure to cope with the demands of modern society, from intemperance, crime, and sexual deviancy to chronic poverty or failure in school.

In Harry Perkins's heredity course, Goddard's theory of feeblemindedness was well integrated into the study of human hereditary "defects." The "Eugenics" section of Newman's textbook surveyed the latest research on human heredity, illustrated in pedigrees of families bearing such "peculiarities" or "abnormalities" as cataracts, polydactylism (extra digits), hemophilia, and Huntington's chorea. A number of Goddard's charts on families bearing the usual repertoire of maladies (feeblemindedness, epilepsy, etc.) that required institutionalization were discussed, along with studies of "competent officials in the employ of insane hospitals," which demonstrated the apparent recessive nature of a variety of mental disorders. While some of Newman's chapters presented strongly *hereditarian* views of human nature, the *interactionist* view of heredity and environment prevails in the other chapters, echoing the sentiments and warnings of J. Arthur Thomson a dozen years before. "Eugenics and Euthenics" by Paul Popenoe and Roswell H. Johnson, for example, restated the importance of recognizing that the germplasm is responsible only for "predisposition" to health or disease and argued that a program of environmental improvement (euthenics) must accompany initiatives for biological improvement of a race (meaning its efficient adaptation to a particular environment): "[T]he best inherited constitution must have a fair chance. And what has been found here as a physical character, would probably hold in even greater degree for a mental character. All that man inherits is the capacity to develop along a certain line under the influence of proper stimuli, food, and exercise."[59]

Discussions of immigration policies in Newman's *Readings* and in other college texts of the period targeted the allegedly inherited "predispositions" to prostitution, tuberculosis, mental defect, eye diseases, and the like and suggested examinations and screening of the family histories of prospective immigrants to prevent such "defective germplasm" from entering the country. While specific groups were not overtly targeted for exclusion in the early editions of these texts, discriminatory immigration policies were tacitly supported. According to H. E. Walter's "Human Conservation," for example, officials granting visas ought to know whether a prospective immigrant "comes from a race of people which, through chronic shiftlessness or lack of initiative, have always carried light purses."[60]

The final chapter of Newman's *Readings*, Caleb Williams Saleeby's "The

Promise of Race Culture," from *Parenthood and Race Culture* (1909), urged caution in misuse of eugenics and emphasized the value of human diversity, the maintenance of human variability as essential to race improvement, and the mutual goals of eugenics and Christianity: "Let it be asserted most emphatically that, if there is anything in the world which eugenics or race culture does *not* promise or desire, it is the production of a uniform type of man. . . . To aim at the suppression of variation, therefore on supposed eugenic grounds (which would be involved in aiming at any uniform type of mankind) would be to aim at destroying the necessary condition of all racial progress."[61] Saleeby used the words of Jesus to demonstrate the eugenic appeal to enlightened Protestants: "I have come that ye may have life, and that ye may have it more abundantly." According to Saleeby, eugenics was the modern expression of Christian purpose: "Progress I define as the emergence and increasing dominance of mind. Of progress thus conceived, man is the highest fruit thereto. He is also the appointed agent and eugenics is his instrument." Perkins had been familiar with Saleeby's work, had well-developed missionary interests of his own, and would embrace the contributions of religious leaders, such as Albert Edward Wiggam, to the eugenics movement.[62]

Perkins followed the general presentation of eugenics of Newman, Castle, Guyer, and Popenoe, whose texts became important sources for the Eugenics Survey. Yet the flood of books, monographs, and popular literature on eugenics provided additional source material for Perkins's students. *The Scientific Papers of the Second International Congress of Eugenics* (1923) provided a diverse array of new research in genetics and eugenics in two substantial volumes, and the *Journal of Heredity* kept Perkins abreast of the latest developments in these fields. The Eugenics Research Association at Cold Spring Harbor and the newly formed American Eugenics Association (1923) provided colleges with general and specific studies on human heredity, eugenics, and their role in public affairs. Because the majority of this research came from academic biologists and medical experts, Perkins would have been little concerned with its legitimacy or its appropriateness in his zoology instruction.

Among all the sources available to Perkins, studies in rural eugenics became most interesting to Perkins and his Vermont students. Studies in rural eugenics rested on the belief that recessive genes, like Goddard's "feeblemindedness gene" and many other hypothetical genes for mental disorders, explained the apparent "life incompetence" and "peculiarities" of isolated and inbred families—the mountain folk of the Appalachians or inhabitants of so-called pockets of degeneracy—familiar figures in the early-twentieth-century popular imagination. The rural poor, once targets of home missionary workers and social reformers of the nineteenth century, became "field populations" for eugenicists studying the transmission of feeblemindedness and other forms of mental incompetence. *The Kallikak Family* (1912) by Henry H.

Goddard, *The Hill Folk* by Charles Davenport, and *The Nam Family: A Study in Cacogenics* (1912) by Arthur Estabrook and Charles Davenport, launched the new genre of literature on rural degeneracy, based on genealogical studies of the rural poor in the midwestern, New England, and southern states.[63]

Families vulnerable to such investigation were poor and socially ostracized and lived outside the accepted moral or social conventions of middle-class America. Their involvement with public charities or corrections could be traced in town and state records over successive generations. Evidence of alleged "delinquency, dependency, and mental defect" (known as the 3 D's) were plotted on pedigree charts to demonstrate recurring patterns of feeble-mindedness, insanity, and a variety of asocial tendencies in family lines. While the family studies initiated a discourse on the genetic sources of social problems, their influence lay in the *association* made between family size, family history, and public expense.

Arthur Estabrook's studies of rural degeneracy, in particular, inspired early eugenics work in Vermont. Estabrook popularized the concept of "cacogenics," the concentration of bad germplasm in poor, inbred, socially isolated and illiterate families, and built his career on studies of cacogenic families. His most famous study, *The Jukes in 1915*, had traced three generations of descendants of a New York family that had been immortalized in William Dugdale's 1877 study, *The Jukes*. Whereas Dugdale had used the Jukes to urge social reforms that would break the cycle of social rejection and poverty, Estabrook attributed their problems to inherited feeblemindedness and innate personality disorders. From pedigrees and records of the New York Department of Charity and Corrections, Estabrook revealed that the Jukes had not only been very prolific, but they had also cost the state of New York a lot of money. The problems of social ostracism and the lack of rehabilitation programs that Dugdale had used the family to exemplify, Estabrook simply incorporated into his tautology. The Jukes, he assumed, originated from social rejects or wayward types, whose inherited defectiveness made them unsuitable mates for the intelligent, ambitious, and principled. Subsequently, they married their own kind, and defective genes accumulated in their descendants. Juxtaposed with a rhetoric of the modern need for a more intelligent, socially minded citizenry and alarm over the declining size of middle- and upper-class families, the rural eugenics literature reduced the complexities of family life and public welfare into a problem of economics and reproductive control. The histories of these families, thus decontextualized, encouraged further discrimination of families caught in the cycle of poverty, social rejection, and loss of opportunity.[64]

While Perkins's heredity course provided students with a biological perspective on mental health and family life and the methods to investigate genetic predispositions in families and selected populations, students enrolled in Professor Asa Gifford's philosophy and psychology courses reflected on the social and ethical dimensions of normal and abnormal mental development. In "Social Ethics" the student became acquainted with "social maladjustments of modern society" and critically studied the "various practical means of applying psychological knowledge and ethical principles to the regulation of social life in its various phases." Problems in "the regulation of family life, industrial relations, voluntary associations, political activities, public health, delinquency, and crime" were addressed in relation to the "ideals of a harmonious and progressive community and national life and a freely developed individuality." In Gifford's physiological psychology class students learned the neurological basis for normal and abnormal behavior, and in his advanced course, social psychology, they studied "the relation of human traits to social tendencies and developments." A eugenic consciousness was cultivated in this course as students related individual achievement to "social environment" and examined "the manner in which individuals and smaller groups influence the life and development of communities."[65] Gifford and Perkins continued the coherence and humanism of the Arts and Sciences curriculum, while applying the expertise of their respective fields to practical problems. By projecting their investigations into the community they translated theories into public service, as the humanistic response to Benton's directive to "make the waste places of the state blossom like the rose." Gifford, however, had been more directly involved in public outreach than Perkins had, and had become a recognized leader in social reforms concerning families and children. Perkins's opportunity for leadership in this endeavor was on the horizon.

The Rebirth of Perkins's Zoological Laboratory as a Eugenics Field Station

From his heredity course, a number of Professor Perkins's students were inspired to continue their study of human inheritance in the context of Zoology 6, "Independent Investigations." Eager as always to encourage original, independent work, Perkins wrote to Charles Davenport, the top-ranking expert in American human genetics, to enlist his advice on the projects his students had chosen. Perkins's students had shown an interest in eye color, colorblindness, height and body structure, family studies of inmates at local orphanages, and interracial marriages (which Perkins felt was "a purely library alcove proposition"). Davenport made a number of pertinent suggestions on all but the topic of interracial marriage, which is curious in light of his own interest in the topic. With regard to the proposed studies of family histories of orphans, Davenport replied that such a project would "reveal very interesting data of great social, if not biological moment."[66] He encouraged Perkins's students to pursue their interests in human heredity and eugenics further at Cold Spring Harbor. Thus began a professional association between Harry Perkins and Charles Davenport that would, over the next seven years, have momentous consequences for Vermont.

Quite possibly, Professor Perkins could have confined his involvement with eugenics to the zoology classroom, but, he later explained, he found himself "lacking definite information about Vermont families. . . . It was all very well to bring forth the results of studies on the Jukes, Kallikaks, Nams, and other graphic examples of degeneracy and, by contrast the generations of notables among the Jonathan Edwards and Hirschoff families; but Vermont students wanted Vermont facts."[67] In a subsequent letter concerning Perkins's initial inquiries, Davenport called attention to a most disturbing Vermont fact: "Did you know, that in the study of defects found in drafted men, Vermont stood at or near the top of the list as having precisely or nearly the highest defect rate for quite a series of defects?"[68] (See fig. 1.5.)

In fact, Vermont leaders had been well aware of the draft board results and used them to promote public health programs and improve medical and dental services, especially for children. But its explicitly eugenic implications had not figured directly into their discussions. Draft board rejections had been invoked by eugenicists since the Boer War as an indicator of deterioration of the national "stocks," but when applied to Vermonters, a people whose record of military achievement in every other war was one of its greatest sources of pride, Perkins paid attention. The draft boards had only reinforced popular perceptions of Vermont's backwardness. "Vermont's reputation suffered," Perkins later reminisced. "This report was getting a rather broad circulation."[69]

Lamarckian theorists would have embraced the nineteenth-century view that rural isolation and struggle against a harsh climate bred self-reliance, ruggedness, and character. But the "modern biological attitude" of the neo-Darwinians could neither support celebrations of Vermonters' struggle with nature as the cause of their virtue nor explain the draft board results. Yet Mendelian genetics and eugenics, as Davenport pointed out, could explain both:

This result I ascribe to the French Canadian constituents of the population which, I had other reasons for believing, to contain an undue proportion of defectives. I wrote to a friend in St. Johnsbury about this and she made some inquiries and concluded that, indeed, there is a large number of gross defects among the French Canadians at that place. Sometimes the population of an island, possibly like Grand Isle in the lake, reveals *a high amount of inbreeding and an unusual percentage of defectives.* Also *mountain valleys,* such as I imagine are to be found in Lamoille County *are places to which the subnormal or*

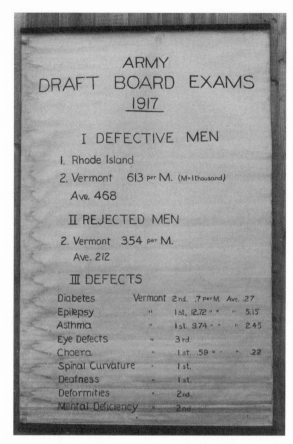

ARMY

DRAFT BOARD EXAMS

1917

I DEFECTIVE MEN

1. Rhode Island

2. Vermont   613 per M. (M=1 thousand)

    Ave. 468

II REJECTED MEN

2. Vermont   354 per M.

    Ave. 212

III DEFECTS

Diabetes	Vermont	2 nd.	.7 per M	Ave.	.27
Epilepsy	"	1 st,	12.72 " "	"	5.15
Asthma	"	1 st.	9.74 " "	"	2.45
Eye Defects	"	3 rd.			
Choera	"	1 st.	.59 " "	"	.22
Spinal Curvature	"	1 st.			
Deafness	"	1 st.			
Deformities	"	2 nd.			
Mental Deficiency	"	2 nd.			

1.5 Harry Perkins prepared this chart showing Vermont's problem at the draft boards in 1925 or 1926 to promote the need for eugenics research and eugenics solutions.
George H. Perkins Papers, University of Vermont Archives. Courtesy Special Collections Department, University of Vermont Library.

unsocial have retreated and produced communities characterized by mental or temperamental defects.[70] (emphasis mine)

Davenport's linkage of the inferiority of Vermont draftees registered a popular perception within a neo-Darwinian framework. To view French Canadians through the same eugenic lenses harmonized with popular Yankee perceptions of their clannishness and inferior intelligence. Davenport's connection convinced Perkins that the connection between rural poverty and the high rate of Vermont "defects" was a simple problem of cacogenics—the concentration of bad heredity through interbreeding among "defectives." Perkins translated his anxieties over Vermont's alleged deterioration into a student research problem. He sent an interested student, Jennie Schneller, to Cold Spring Harbor in 1924 to investigate the Vermont draft board data and subsequently turned the draft board problem into a class project.[71]

The "historic moment" when Perkins realized the potential for his own original eugenics research arrived in 1924. Perkins later recalled the epiphany that inspired his formation of the Eugenics Survey of Vermont:

> . . . A most suggestive, thought-provoking pedigree chart came to [my] notice. Prepared by a *State Department of Welfare investigator*, it set forth a large proportion of *defective, delinquent, and dependent* individuals in a family of which one or two persons had found their way into a state institution. Would it not be valuable to produce other charts, not only of families in which the three "d's" were the most prevalent characteristics but in the higher types of families in which contributions to the upbuilding of the state and her institutions were conspicuous and numerous?[72] (emphasis mine)

While the draft board results offered a rationale and the eugenics literature suggested a methodology, the Vermont Department of Public Welfare provided the point of entry and the point of departure for Perkins's eugenics field studies of Vermonters. In 1925, Perkins made his bid to lead this research through organizing a eugenics society, modeled on those in other universities. As an adjunct to his department, it could serve as an "experimental field station" to study the "Vermont facts" of family life, identify the sources of Vermont's alleged degeneracy, and offer "scientific" solutions to improving the genetic health of the Vermont population. Such an enterprise would enable Professor Perkins to conduct socially relevant and "practical" research and apply his professional expertise to important local issues to advance his reputation. Perhaps he too could achieve the celebrated reputation of his father in the university and the state and keep his mother's spirit of social reform alive. Eugenics was not without criticism from scientists and non-scientists in the 1920s. But neither, incidentally, was evolution. Perkins had witnessed over forty years of religious and scientific opposition to Darwinism, which had motivated the research to produce a consensus. There was no reason for Perkins to suspect eugenics would be any different.

Perkins's utopian vision of merging eugenics with progressive social reform in Vermont would have remained simply a pipe dream without the support of a constituency of sympathetic Vermont leaders. The new university president, Guy W. Bailey, heartily endorsed Perkins's initiative and assisted him behind the scenes to secure the necessary support. The practical difficulties of producing charts of allegedly defective Vermont families from institutional records would require the permission and cooperation of private social agencies and state institutions. While Perkins took the initiative to use his talents, his vision, and his connections to lead the quest for a "eugenic Vermont," the incentives for such an endeavor and the infrastructure to support it had evolved in other contexts outside the domain of academic biology.

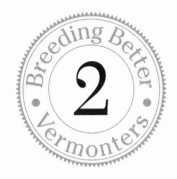

Foundations for a
Eugenic Survey of Vermont,
1890–1925

> Until recently most Vermonters had lived in the happy illusion
> that their state had no child welfare problems, that children were
> well cared for in their homes except for a few orphans who were
> adequately provided for in its institutions. Even before the influ-
> enza epidemic, however, the belief that all was well with Vermont
> children was beginning to be questioned.
>
> **—L. Josephine Webster, Vermont Children's Aid Society**

The connection of social factors with heredity was not new in Vermont and
did not originate with Harry Perkins. Nor did the search for "degenerate
families." Yet a decade prior to the birth of the Eugenics Survey of Vermont
or a decade afterward the idea of constructing genealogies of Vermont's "degenerate families" would have been inconceivable. Eugenics in Vermont was
by no means inevitable. Many obstacles—cultural, historical, and political—
stood in the way of a eugenics program for the state, not the least of which
was Vermont's sense of autonomy and its unwillingness to follow the trends in
the big cities. Neither the urban problems of large-scale foreign immigration
and the social blight of industrial slums nor the Progressive concern with

women's rights, child labor, and the human abuses of rampant capitalism seemed directly relevant to Vermont's interests or problems. Vermonters frequently made a virtue of their isolation from such outside influences and of their ability to take care of their own problems. Ironically, it was this tradition of self-reliance and Vermonters' pride in it that ultimately drove the comprehensive eugenics program of the state.

Vermont's apparent unique character rested on its traditional rural geography and economy and town-based politics, a way of life that many Americans associated with the Jeffersonian agrarian America of the past—a refuge from the alienation and mechanization associated with modern industrial progress. Yet the tension between a nostalgic identity and the demands of the modern age, when interpreted against Vermont's vision of its own heroic role in the history of the republic, became a growing source of discomfort after the turn of the century. Two themes in the literature of the centennial era (1890–1910) defined Vermont and Vermonters—a statehood that arose from a struggle for its integrity as an independent republic and its continual production of men and women of tough moral fiber, intelligence, and leadership, who played key roles in every major event in American history, from the War of Independence to the abolition of slavery and the settlement of the American frontier. It was within this traditional, mythical image of the state and its people that eugenic studies of Vermonters took place.

The Facts of Demography:
Population Change or Population Anxiety?

In the early twentieth century many Americans had begun to think in terms of "race betterment" and to worry about "race suicide." Theodore Roosevelt had helped to popularize the latter formula through public commentary and his own writings on eugenics. Roosevelt had used the term to call attention to the central importance of conserving the "American family" at a time when Anglo-Americans were having, on the average, fewer children. The race suicide metaphor became a unifying concept to link public discourses on the social and financial costs of crime, poverty, and public health to the changing values and ethnic makeup of the nation.[1] The "closing of the frontier," the growth and industrialization of cities with their associated health and social problems, continued immigration of Europeans and Asians (once a welcome source of labor), the "woman question" and the agitation of feminists for political and legal equality, all conspired to kindle population anxieties and concern over the future of the nation. Yet national awareness of "race suicide" was not a defining theme of discussions of the Vermont population.

In other regions of the United States, the post–World War I years brought huge demographic changes. Immigrants from eastern and southern Europe poured in, adding to the changing character of urban life caused by an equally large-scale internal migration from country to city. African Americans were migrating from southern rural areas to large cities in the North in search of economic opportunities. Such changes fueled racial prejudice, nativistic sentiment, and white Anglo-Saxon Protestant anxiety over their declining dominance in the American population. Many Vermonters shared these sentiments. Vermont senator William Paul Dillingham, for example, spearheaded the enactment of stricter immigration restrictions to restore the nineteenth-century ethnic composition of the country. In 1921, Vermont native son Calvin Coolidge openly publicized his concern that America had become a "dumping ground" for the "wrong kind" of immigrants and signed into law the Immigration Restriction Act of 1924 when he became president. Most Vermonters, despite their pride in their role as leaders in the emancipation of slaves, ignored injustices to African Americans in southern states, and some actively supported the persecution of racial minorities by the Ku Klux Klan.[2]

Despite America's changing demography, the Vermont population had in fact remained relatively stable in both size and ethnic or racial composition. The state remained 71 percent native-born Yankee, and the immigration of Irish, French Canadians, English, Italians, and Germans had not dramatically changed since the decades following the Civil War. Native American presence in Vermont communities was not formally acknowledged, and Asians and African Americans were most often noted for their absence or rare appearance in Vermont communities. The anxieties of politicians at the federal level over the ethnic composition of the American population and the reinforcement of those fears by eugenicists' analyses of defects among various immigrant groups may have sensitized Vermont leaders to their own ethnic diversity.[3] Yet the demographic composition of the state between 1890 and 1920 suggests both continuity and stability in the racial and ethnic diversity of the Vermont population. Furthermore, Vermont had actually shown a decline in total population between 1910 and 1920.

Within Vermont, however, the internal redistribution of the population and its changing complexion had profound implications for state identity when interpreted against the backdrop of the state's celebrated heritage. Throughout the nineteenth century, Vermont leaders had been concerned over the abandonment of rural farms and small villages by the younger generation, eager for the economic and social opportunities in the cities and the midwestern states. Vermonters' pride in the prosperity and achievements of their emigrant native sons fueled anxiety that those who stayed behind had lacked the initiative, courage, or talent of those who had left for greener pastures. Vermont census figures from 1890 to 1920 revealed a decline in the working age group (15 to 40 years old) and a corresponding increase in senior citizens. Demographics also revealed an unprecedented shift of the Vermont population from the "rural" to the "non-rural" category. Agricultural towns, particularly those along the Green Mountains, the backbone of the state, were losing wealth and population, while Chittenden, Washington, and Windsor counties, where urban centers were located, were growing and prospering.[4] Because the ruggedness of the hillside farms in the Green Mountains had defined Vermont's character and people, these findings were cause for concern. The loss of community infrastructure associated with severely depopulated towns and the gradual replacement of the descendants of the Yankee settlers with "foreign" Catholic immigrants, primarily French Canadians from Quebec, placed Vermont's population anxieties within a local, cultural context.

French Canadians formed the largest non-Yankee element in the state as a result of their gradual and sustained immigration from Quebec. At the turn of the century, French Canadians were ever scarcely mentioned in Vermont literature without invoking their role in the early history of the state. French Canadians and their Indian (Abenaki) allies were portrayed as the early colonial settlers' ancient foe, whose assaults they had endured and who had to be defeated in order to create the Republic of Vermont. Vermont poet and historian Rowland E. Robinson popularized this legend in the 1890s. Robinson's *Vermont: A Study of Independence* (1892), for example, depicted Vermont as "the highway of war" and the "battleground in the wilderness" in the French and Indian Wars, where early settlers trying to make a home on the land became the innocent victims, either massacred or captured by the Abenaki, under French command, and taken to Montreal for ransom. The descendants of the French Canadians who settled in Vermont, after moving back and forth across the border for seasonal work, represented, in Robinson's analysis, an "insidious and continuous invasion" of the remnants of a defeated enemy. While he appreciated the fact that many of them rivaled the Yankee in ruggedness and willingness to improve the farms they acquired, their homes nevertheless "looked and smelled as if they had been transplanted from Canada with their owners." The following passage of Robinson's depiction of nineteenth-century French Canadian immigrants served as a defining narrative for studies of some French Canadian families by the Eugenics Survey of Vermont:

> For years the state was infested with an inferior class of people, who plied the vocation of professional beggars. They made regular trips through the country in bands consisting of one or more families, with horses, carts, and ricketty wagons, and a retinue of curs, soliciting alms of pork, potatoes, and breadstuffs at every farmhouse they came to, and pilfering when opportunity offered. In large towns there were depots where the proceeds of their beggary and theft were

disposed of. They were an abominable crew of vagabonds, robust, lazy men and boys, slatternly women with litters of filthy brats, and all as detestable as they were uninteresting. They worked their beats successfully, till their pitiful tales of sickness, burnings-out, and journeyings to friends in distant towns worn threadbare, and then they gradually disappeared, no one knows whither.[5]

While the underlying themes of rootlessness, speculation for personal gain, and disappearance may have been an unconscious projection of the American anxieties of the Gilded Age, Robinson also worried about the cultural implications of French Canadian assimilation in Vermont. He wondered where French Canadian Vermonters placed their true allegiance and what impact their growing presence would have on the character of the state. From his perspective, Catholicism, when practiced, represented an attempt on the part of the Catholic priesthood to undermine the social fabric of Vermont Protestant communities. When not practiced, the French Canadian became part of the unchurched, unsettled population and therefore highly suspect. "What this leaven may finally work in the Protestant mass with which it has become incorporated," Robinson reflected, "is a question that demands more attention than it has received. The character of these people is not as to inspire the highest hope for the future of Vermont, if they should become a numerous part of the population. The affiliation with Anglo-Americans of a race so different in traits, in traditions, and in religion must necessarily be slow, and may never be complete."[6] Harry Perkins would eventually attend to this question, discover some of the "roving bands" that Robinson believed had disappeared, and turn Robinson's narratives into his own eugenic ones.

Not all Vermonters shared Robinson's pessimism over the "immigrant leaven." After the turn of the century the consequences of the loss of community infrastructure in poor, sparsely populated areas became a larger concern. Some observers made explicit connections between rural depopulation, the failure to maintain churches and schools, and the evident social and moral decay of affected communities. The abandoned farms, the empty churches, the closed academies and schools—all symbolized neglect and a loss of authority of the institutions that conveyed Vermont traditions and values. Unschooled and unchurched, some rural communities had lost the means to cultivate the mind and the character, essential to the health and prosperity of their coming citizens. Whether the perceived human degradation resulted from a loss of revenue or a loss of leadership, the problem commanded the attention of rural sociologists, economists, and ministers, who investigated the conditions of rural decline in Vermont and other New England towns, published their findings, and offered solutions.

Vermont-born minister Wilbert E. Anderson, for example, had studied at Oberlin College and returned to Vermont with an interest in rural sociology and modern views of the role of the Protestant ministry. After preaching in Stowe for a few years he turned to scholarly study of the rural exodus. In *The Country Town: A Study of Rural Evolution* (1906), an interesting synthesis of neo-Darwinism, William James's psychology, rural sociology, and Vermont demographic data, Anderson argued that the problem of rural decline would resolve itself over time by a biocultural evolution. The "individual man," whose physical strength and innate tolerance of solitude had enabled him to make a home in the wilderness, would give way to the "social man," whose greater intellect and more highly developed cooperative instincts were suited to the modern age. Scientific, practical education would cultivate the "rural mind" in this direction, and the transformation of country churches into community social centers would develop a moral social consciousness. Anderson was optimistic about the gradual infusion of foreign immigrants in rural Vermont. He predicted that they would assimilate successfully in country towns that offered modern social and civic opportunities and that "enough of the original population will remain in the country to set a wholesome standard of life, to perpetuate ancient ideals, and to dominate the incoming races."[7]

Another Vermont minister, Charles Otis Gill, actually put such an idea into practice in one Vermont town, which had not seen a minister in twenty years. By refashioning the church into a community social institution with a religious and moral center, he claimed to have transformed the town from a place of vice and loose living into a socially responsible, vital community. His resulting publications, *The Country Church: The Decline of Its Influence and the Remedy* (1913) and *Six Thousand Country Churches* (1920), in collaboration with conservationist Gifford Pinchot, became important sources for the Eugenics Survey of Vermont.[8]

Economic Transition and Rural Renewal

At the turn of the century, agriculture in Vermont had undergone a series of adjustments as part of the modernizing process. Following the time frames laid out by Harold Fisher Wilson in his pioneering study, *The Hill Country of Northern New England: Its Social and Economic History in the Nineteenth and Twentieth Centuries*, the late nineteenth century was the "winter" of Vermont agriculture. During Wilson's "winter" (1870–1900), Vermont experienced a decline in agricultural prosperity and many farms on "marginal" land were abandoned. After 1900, Wilson's "spring," many Vermont farmers, with the support of agricultural organizations and encouragement by the state, modernized their dairy operations and profited from diversification. Meat, fruit, and vegetable production; forest products; and hosting summer visitors reinvigorated the rural economy in many parts of Vermont after the turn of the century. Farmers who had made Wilson's transition into spring prospered. Recognized as adaptable and productive, these newly prosperous farmers provided a contrast to others, who by choice or necessity sustained the independent, self-contained, traditional ways of farming.

The contrast in circumstances between the adaptable spring farmers and the conservative, independent winter farmers was recapitulated at the town level in the early twentieth century. Declining property values in towns that were losing wealth and population contributed to an escalation in property tax rates. The tax inequities further crippled the independent hillside farmers in those areas, who had to contribute larger portions of their meager incomes to support town schools, roads, and charity as required by law. The dramatic reduction in the number of working farms in the majority of Vermont towns, a decline in population in the majority of rural towns, and a corresponding increase in the size and productivity of farms in fertile, easily mechanized, accessible areas required a new definition of Vermont self-sufficiency as well. By 1930 only 6 percent of Vermont farms were the self-sufficient variety that had, for over a century, defined the character of the state and its people in the popular imagination.[9]

Vermont's rural exodus and the resulting economic plight of farmers in the winter of the late nineteenth century was part of a national trend that had worried national and state leaders throughout the Progressive era. The country life movement had developed out of this concern and a desire to improve the conditions of farm life and thereby restore the Jeffersonian vision of an agrarian America. Scientific management of agriculture through extension services, the Grange, and agricultural education promised to improve efficiency of production, while efforts to upgrade rural education, recreation, and civic life would improve the quality of life in the country. Such reforms, country life proponents argued, would encourage the ambitious and well-educated to remain or return to rural life and replenish the pioneer stocks that had made the nation great. Ministers, rural sociologists, scientists, and conservationists pressed for rural reform. Theodore Roosevelt convened a National Commission on Country Life in 1908 to study the associated problems of conservation of human resources and the quality of agricultural life. Its recommendations appealed to many progressive intellectuals and state leaders in Vermont. Vermont may have been the only state that achieved a formal, explicit connection between eugenics and the country life movement. Yet eugenicists and country life advocates often found common ground in the application of the principles of conservation and "wise use" to human resources. Many well-known conservationists, like Teddy Roosevelt and Gifford Pinchot, supported both.[10]

Alongside the country life movement, the Vermont Board of Agriculture had been encouraging rural families since the 1890s to supplement their incomes by taking in visitors who enjoyed the nostalgic, bucolic retreat from the stress and industrial blight of modern urban life. The board had been actively promoting Vermont country life in the tourist literature and had assumed the function of selling the "imaginary" Vermont to affluent visitors and potential settlers in the state. Attraction of a "higher class of people" to replace those who had left the state was one goal of tourist promotion. If such visitors became residents, they could restore the rural charm, upgrade the rural culture, and invigorate the rural economy. The expected class of new-comers, attracted to Vermont's natural beauty, would work hard to preserve and cultivate it.[11]

The advertisement of Vermont as a nostalgic retreat into a romantic image of childhood in the country increasingly appealed to many Americans. The tourist economy grew in the 1910s, and after World War I, tourism became an important source of income for the state. Wealthy "outlanders" acquired and developed lakeshore properties for summer retreats, and tourists travel-ing by automobile explored more remote areas of Vermont in the summer months. Outdoor recreation, beautiful "unspoiled" scenery, and Vermont's legendary past appealed to Americans, particularly after World War I. Ver-mont appeared to have preserved a way of life that had been celebrated since the Civil War as "American" and was rapidly retreating in space and time. But given the facts of Vermont agriculture in the 1920s, that disappearing Yankee farmer, the "pioneer" of the American imagination, would have to be *created*. Those Vermonters still living in the old manner in more isolated communities were finding themselves in reduced circumstances, described in terms of "rural subnormalcy" or portrayed as primitive. Families who took advantage of the opportunity to amplify their income by taking in summer visitors had to adjust their homes, their manners, and their appearance to sell the rustic Vermont image, often at considerable inconvenience.[12]

What happened to those who endured within the older rural culture de-spite the decline in their circumstances? What became of those who had sold their land to pay off debts and had to move on? What happened to the chil-dren and grandchildren of those who had sold out a generation earlier? What sort of pressures were brought at the local level, or by interested land devel-opers from other areas, on those who resisted a change in their independent way of life? Certainly some who had abandoned their own bankrupt farms were employed as laborers on profitable farms. Most of them probably found work in businesses or industries in growing town or cities. Others likely became part of the "transient" or "dependent" population, perhaps seeking charity and labeled as "paupers." Those who resisted "progress" and lived be-yond the boundaries of Vermont's new conventions became more vulnerable to the efforts of civil authorities and social reformers to diagnose their needs and deliver them to such "places of refuge" as the reformatories, the poor farms, and institutions for the feebleminded and insane. While some of these people may have been casualties of the agrarian transformation, certainly others, who had always lived a marginal or vagabond existence within the state, appeared even more anachronistic within the context of the more modern Vermont.

Popular literature, professional sources, and government documents of the early twentieth century demonstrate a peculiar ambivalence about the hill farmers, the transient population, and the "unusual" types of people for which Vermont had become known. Romantic admiration of their freedom from social constraints and carefree simplicity was juxtaposed with disdain for their lack of education, poor hygiene, and disregard for the sexual conventions of middle-class America. The sentimental image of the God-fearing, nature-loving farmer, tending his fields and rearing healthy children against a backdrop of Vermont's unspoiled hills and meadows, was too often spoiled by deteriorating or abandoned farms, shabby tenements or shacks on the outskirts of rural villages, and the periodic influx of rowdy, hard-drinking dirt farmers on supply trips into Burlington.

Vermont Traditions of Charity and the "Social Problem Group"

Problems exist only in proportion to the amount of visibility given them, the level of importance attributed to them, and the degree of impotence concerned parties experience as they confront them. By all these measures, charity to the poor, child health and welfare, the rehabilitation of delinquents, and the care of the handicapped had become problems of unprecedented proportion in Vermont during the early twentieth century. Beginning in the 1890s, Vermont leaders and commentators had become increasingly aware of the relationship between the problems of dependency, delinquency, and mental defect (the so-called 3 Ds) and the celebrated character of the Vermont people. When Harry Perkins addressed these problems in his teachings on heredity, he merely superimposed a eugenic explanation on an existing framework of defining, interpreting, and managing the "social problem group" already established by others.

In the second decade of the twentieth century, Vermont civic leaders and progressive reformers began to conduct surveys to assess how efficiently government agencies functioned in managing state services and to evaluate the effectiveness of towns in meeting their obligations to the people. Such studies engendered a growing awareness of the gap between Vermont social realities and Vermonters' "happy illusion" that the state was successfully managing its affairs. The revelations of the "scientific" surveys of Vermont government, public charity, and the education system created an enormous tension between Vermonters' own vision of their state as self-reliant, adaptable, and resourceful and the apparent inadequacy of its institutions to manage the problems of crime, poverty, and disease in the state.

Throughout the nineteenth century, charity to the poor, care of the disabled, and many of the various police powers of the state had been administered at the local level. In 1797, in response to an apparently increasing, mobile poor population, the state legislature had passed a law, stating: "that every town and place in this state shall relieve, support, and maintain their own poor. And the overseers . . . shall relieve, support, and maintain all the poor, lame, blind, sick, and other inhabitants within such town or place, who are not able to maintain themselves . . . provide for them houses, nurses, physicians, and surgeons."[13] Newcomers to a town who either requested charity or appeared likely to need it could be "warned out" at the discretion of the selectmen, a procedure that would relieve the town of its obligation to extend poor relief to outsiders. As more Vermonters had fallen into poverty in the early nineteenth century, towns had collaborated to create poor farms and poorhouses, which quickly became the permanent residences of mentally ill and physically disabled persons who could not be supported by their families. Poor farms and poorhouses also served as temporary refuges or holding areas for the transient poor and hard-luck cases. Abuses of mentally handicapped residents in these places had encouraged the establishment of the Brattleboro Retreat in 1836, a private mental hospital supplemented by state funds, and the State Hospital for the Insane at Waterbury in 1890.[14]

In the mid-nineteenth century the state had begun to assume more responsibility for handicapped children living in poverty. The governor served as their trustee until 1923, when the newly formed Department of Public Welfare assumed this responsibility. After the Civil War reform-minded men and women, often affiliated with church home missionary work, began to organize private charities for orphaned, neglected, or destitute children, providing additional resources to towns on a regional or statewide basis.[15] Concern over the treatment of juvenile offenders led to the establishment of the Vermont Reform School in Vergennes in 1865 (renamed the Vermont Industrial School in 1898). Created independently in response to diverse social concerns, the various state and regional facilities of the nineteenth century were directed, funded, and operated somewhat autonomously. Supervisory boards and "visiting committees" were constituted to review conditions and expenditures, investigate complaints, and consider needs. Referrals to institutions were made on an individual, ad hoc basis. Town authorities, usually overseers of the poor, or other interested parties, referred growing numbers of needy, neglected, or apparently disabled children, "town charges," and "undesirables" to the available institutions. Parents or town selectmen could initiate such placements, and frequently children who were neither delinquent nor mentally deficient were diagnosed as such in order to relieve the town of its responsibility for their care.[16] The gradual shift in responsibility for the supervision and care of the "social problem group" from the towns to state and private institutions and the growing demand for these services contributed to an apparent need to expand the existing facilities or construct new ones. The demand for more institutional space provoked anxiety over the apparently growing population of dependent, delinquent, and disabled persons and the rising costs of their care. Within a single generation, the growth of institutions and their use as a means for towns to fulfill their legal obligation to the poor had created a segregated, concentrated, and visible population of "defective and dependent" Vermonters.

In the 1890s eugenic thinking began to filter into Vermont philanthropic organizations through the publications of professional organizations involved in corrections, child welfare, and mental health. The annual reports of the Home for Destitute Children (HDC) in Burlington, for example, reflect the 1890s shift in emphasis from care and cure to cause and prevention. In 1893 the HDC was portrayed as a city of refuge "to save children from a life of ignorance, misery, and sin, and place them where they can receive Christian nurture."[17] Beginning in 1895 the annual reports showed a greater concern over "adult persons of feeble-mind, or imbeciles," who were perceived to be a danger to public safety when "at large" in the community. In 1899, HDC president Sarah Torrey recast their mission in modern terms: "We look to the transformation of the weak, helpless and unfit into the strong, helpful and efficient . . . and we aim to choke off at its fountain source some of the flood of pauperism, imbecility, and vice, and in this way be a blessing to our beloved State and to the world."[18]

Social reform groups also organized legislative committees to bring their agendas before the state legislature in the interest of legal reform of public services. In 1897, when Sarah Torrey urged the state to provide "a place of refuge" for "adult indigent imbecile women of child-bearing age," she drew support from a report of the National Conference of Charities and Corrections, which had presented "startling statistics" indicating that feeblemindedness was inherited, largely through the mother: "It seems certain that from this class come many recruits for the great army of illegitimate children, and of criminals, inebriates, and prostitutes. The article clearly shows most convincingly the necessity for State custodial care of the feebleminded."[19]

In 1912 the state of Vermont established the State School for the Feebleminded at Brandon, Vermont. Not surprisingly, the available spaces filled rapidly. The state school had a considerable waiting list in a very few years as increasing numbers of children of indigent parents were categorized as "feebleminded." The superintendents of Brandon had difficulty at times restricting the use of this facility to those for whom it was intended.[20]

The same year that the State School for the Feebleminded opened, the Vermont legislature passed a bill, "An Act to Authorize and Provide for the Sterilization of Imbeciles, Feeble-minded and Insane Persons, Rapists, Confirmed Criminals, and Other Defectives," on the recommendation of outgoing governor John A. Mead, a physician and enthusiast of modernization. The bill was vetoed by Governor Allen Fletcher, on the advice of his attorney-general, R. A. Brown, who anticipated the unconstitutionality of the statute.[21] In fact nearly all of the seventeen laws passed in other states prior to World War I were repealed or struck down by the courts. This first wave of American interest in sterilization had originated in the medical community, particularly among physicians working in public institutions, who had experimented with the procedure as a form of therapy for criminals and feebleminded children. President Theodore Roosevelt's writings on eugenics, the favorable editorials in *Scientific American* concerning sterilization, and considerable support for eugenic sterilization among professional social workers engaged in charities and corrections services lent a certain legitimacy to what had heretofore been viewed as a spartan approach to social reform.[22]

"The Evil That Lurks in These Hamlets in the Hills"

Vermont was the last of the eastern states to organize a state chapter of the National Conference of Charities and Corrections. In January 1916 forty interested citizens met in Burlington to formally establish one. Its stated purpose was "to unite the voluntary efforts of all who are interested in charitable, correctional, and welfare work of the state and to promote such work by agitation and discussion." Annual conferences provided a forum for discussion of relevant and timely topics, where attendees learned of welfare work in Vermont and other states, shared their experiences, and cooperated to bring social welfare policy in the state in line with national standards. Publication and dissemination of their proceedings would inform the public of the social problems that demanded reform. A crucially important function of the new organization was to study existing social legislation and recommend reforms. The case studies and surveys brought before the conference began a process of rendering the complex problems of families living in poverty into two root causes: feeblemindedness and vice. From the outset, this discourse was directly linked to Vermonters' failure to protect the "state's greatest asset," its children.[23]

The Vermont Conference of Charities and Corrections (VCCC) chose the theme "The Dependent Child" for its second annual meeting (January 1917). Norwich University professor of political science K. R. B. Flint brought the findings from his statewide survey of poor relief before the conference and

urged a complete reform of the current system. Professor Flint had organized the Institute of Municipal Affairs at Norwich and served as its director.
His newly published study, *Poor Relief in Vermont*, reflected his philosophy
of government efficiency through municipal planning and his belief in prevention of human misery through attacking its causes. Moreover, Flint supported eugenic solutions; *Poor Relief in Vermont* became a key source for the
Eugenics Survey throughout its existence.[24]

Poor Relief in Vermont defined the problem with a detailed discussion of
the history and implementation of the current system of the poor laws in Vermont. To study the effects of the traditional system, Flint had surveyed all the
overseers of the poor, visited the poorhouses and poor farms, and compiled
statistics. From this survey, he constructed a profile of the current town-
based system of poor relief, showing it to be expensive, primitive, unhealthy,
and inhumane. He created a taxonomy of dependency, which distinguished
between the deserving and undeserving recipients of charity. Poverty was not
pauperism, Flint explained. The former was due to temporary loss of "neces-
saries"; the latter was characterized by shiftlessness and lack of initiative.
Paupers habitually sought public charity or had grown so accustomed to receiving it that they had fallen into perpetual dependence. Those who by misfortune could not support themselves (including abandoned teenage mothers and widows) deserved help. Mothers' Aid allowances should be granted
to prevent the breaking up of kinship groups. The handicapped, the mentally
ill and feebleminded, the elderly without savings, and those suffering from
chronic diseases such as tuberculosis, whose families were unable to support
them, also deserved public support. Their needs were best met in specialized
institutions. Flint was disturbed to find children, tuberculosis patients, syphi-
litics, and "feebleminded" persons collected together into poorhouses and
poor farms. Children especially should not be exposed to the dangers of
disease and vice found among inmates in poorhouses. The state, he argued,
should provide appropriate institutions for each problem in order to administer to the diverse needs of the dependent population. The feebleminded,
Flint contended, could be educated to some level, and as feeblemindedness
was presumably hereditary, "sterilization or segregation of the feebleminded
may gradually eliminate their kind."[25]

Flint's revelations of the dangers to children living under Vermont's outdated poor relief system resonated with the reports of children's charities, the
state Board of Health, and the superintendents of the Vermont Industrial
School and the School for the Feebleminded. Incidents of incest and illegiti-
macy, domestic violence, alcoholism, and entire families infected with syphilis supported contentions that "defectives breed defectives" and that their
habit of doing so at such an alarming rate was responsible for the rise in delinquency, the spread of disease, and the growing burden on the taxpayer for

poor relief. From the chorus of complaints against "incompetent" and "immoral" parents emerged a consensus that the modern state must serve as the ultimate guardian of children's health and future. VCCC president W. J. Van Patten agreed with Flint that "Vermont has been very backward" in meeting its obligations to its children. He contributed several more narratives of child abuse to the caldron of festering degeneracy that reformers had discovered and urged a more rigorous implementation of the child welfare law passed in 1915.

The 1915 child welfare law, Act 92, legally defined the children of the social problem group and established legal procedures for their rescue. By law, the "dependent and neglected child" was a child under sixteen years of age "who is dependent upon the public for support; or who is homeless, destitute, or abandoned; or who begs or receives alms; or who is found living in a house of ill fame or with a vicious or disreputable person; or whose home by reason of neglect, cruelty, or depravity on the part of his parents, guardian or other person in whose care he may be, is in an unfit place for said child, or whose environment is such to warrant the state, in the interests of the child, in assuming guardianship."[26]

The Juvenile Court Law of 1912 had been enacted to prevent juvenile delinquents from being tried as criminals. The 1915 definition of the "delinquent child" in Act 92 gave local authorities and private citizens who wished to rid their communities of youthful offenders considerable latitude to do so:

> The words "delinquent child" shall, for the purposes of this act, include a child under sixteen years of age who violates a law of this state or a city or village ordinance; or who is incorrigible; or who is a persistent truant from school; or who associates with criminals; or vicious or immoral persons; or who is growing up in idleness or crime; or who wanders about in the streets at night time; or who frequents, visits, or is found in a disorderly house, house of ill-fame, saloon, barroom or a place where a gambling device is operated; or who uses obscene, vulgar, profane or indecent language, or is guilty of immoral conduct.[27]

According to Act 92, any "reputable person" could petition the court to investigate alleged incidents of child neglect, abuse, or delinquency. Municipal courts or justices of the peace, at their discretion, would then charge local probation officers to investigate such cases. Members of the VCCC welcomed these progressive laws. Prior to 1915, Van Patten noted, "the neglected child was *left to the mercy of its parents* or guardians *unless rescued* by private individuals. The delinquent child was tried and sentenced as a criminal"[28] (emphasis mine).

In Van Patten's view, however, many helpless children still remained out of reach of would-be rescuers and at the mercy of "immoral" or abusive parents.

Van Patten told of a family of four children, a boy of fifteen, two girls, ages thirteen and nine, and a baby. "The mother is a half-witted woman and the father an ugly brute. Family lives in a logging camp of one room about 12 feet square. The walls are caked with dirt and there is practically no furniture. Children sleep in piles of rags on the floor." Yet even with the help of the current child protection law, well-meaning neighbors were powerless to help these children, whose future lay in peril:

> Father is known to be selling cider but neighbors are afraid to testify against him as he avenged former interferences in his affairs by burning their barns and poisoning their livestock. He is exceedingly cruel to the children, kicking them and beating them. A rough crowd of men hang around the place drinking and carousing and one of these men has committed rape upon both of the young girls. One of the girls has also been assaulted by her older brother. Repeated efforts have been made to do something for this family, but the father resists any interference and since he provides in a half-way fashion for his children, the selectmen have no right to interfere.

Patten's story illustrated the need for stronger laws and more state support for local officials. But his conclusion made the case for early intervention, before children had been so thoroughly corrupted that there was no hope: "The youngest girl is thought by the school teacher to be a promising child if she had half an opportunity. The oldest boy and girl are undoubtedly feebleminded. Both of these children are already dangerous in the community. The boy is being trained in chicken stealing and small thieving by his father; the girl having already been trained in immorality will soon prove a greater menace."[29]

In 1917, in response to agitation by the VCCC, the state legislature passed a law that ended the practice of keeping children on poor farms, except for short periods and in extreme emergencies. Overseers of the poor were to administer state-supplied Mothers' Aid allowances (in order to preserve and strengthen family units) or arrange for children to be placed in suitable foster homes or in appropriate private or public institutions. The legislature also established the state Board of Charities and Probation to assist towns in this effort and to begin collecting files of children believed to be in need of such services, as was the practice in other states.[30] Because juvenile delinquency was a major concern and because many needy children were found by Vermont courts to be delinquent as well, the secretary of the Board of Charities and Probation would serve in the capacity of state probation officer, converting the former county probation officers to deputy probation officers. Not only did these administrative innovations centralize authority and support local efforts to help or rescue neglected children, they also set a new precedent in which designated agencies and "experts" went forth in search of the social problem group rather than simply responding to cases referred to them from local authorities.[31]

In January 1918 the Vermont Conference of Social Work (heretofore the VCCC) held its third annual conference. W. H. Jeffrey, the first state probation officer, reported the progress of his board in its first six months of operation and further magnified the extent of Vermont's child neglect problem. Jeffrey's cases were not new to this group but added one more voice to the lamentations of Flint, Van Patten, and others over the "evil that lurks in these hamlets in the hills."[32] Yet Jeffrey's cases revealed just how successfully his department had "rescued" children, placing them in foster care or state institutions and charging their parents with child neglect. For example, in the southern part of the state, Jeffrey reported a family of six living in a one-room house of sixteen by eighteen feet: "Inside and outside, the house was filthy, disorderly and shocking. Only two beds and these ragged and dirty provided accommodations for six persons. There was no attempt at privacy, and the fact that a ten and a fifteen-year-old girl were compelled to sleep, robe, and disrobe in the presence of not only the father and mother, but a sixteen year old brother was demoralizing in the extreme." Jeffrey's solution was a total one: "The mother and children were brought into court, and I am pleased to be able to state that the father and the boy George are in the House of Correction, Viola [age 15] is at the School for the Feebleminded at Brandon, Annie [age 10] is at Vergennes [reform school] and Frank, the two year old is still our problem."[33] Jeffrey reported thirty-one child rescues in the first six months, over half of whom were placed at the State School for the Feebleminded and the Vermont Industrial School. From his investigations during this period the Board of Charities and Probation had developed a file of 241 cases of the sort he cited at this conference.[34]

Eugenics and public health movements in America and abroad were synchronized at times and fell into dispute at others. In Vermont they found common ground in their promotion of early diagnosis of defects in children and their conviction that negligent and incompetent parents and insufficient state services were the source of most health and developmental problems. Following Jeffrey's revelations of the horrors of child neglect, Vermont state Board of Health secretary Dr. Charles Dalton reflected on the effects of war and disease on Vermonters and the negligence with which Vermonters had addressed the problems of child health. He announced the surgeon general's report of the high rate of army draft board rejections in Vermont, noting that with early detection and treatment in childhood 90 percent of the conditions, mostly physical ones, could have been prevented. Yet Dalton asserted that the greatest menace to the health of the population and the "efficiency of men" were the "twin vices of alcoholism and immorality." Partly because of the movements of troops during wartime, venereal disease was spreading; he estimated over seven thousand infective cases in Vermont. His department had discovered entire families infected with syphilis, due to their sexual misconduct at home and in the community. Poverty also contributed to the spread of syphilis among children, he explained, as the poor shared clothing, eating utensils, and sleeping arrangements. The spread of gonorrhea among school children in some towns had required public schools to close temporarily. The immorality, ignorance, and negligence of the parents were the source of contagion, in Dalton's view, and children and infants whose mothers were infected during pregnancy were its victims.[35]

Children's Year and the New Guardians of Young Vermont

After World War I, the U.S. Children's Bureau declared 1918–1919 Children's Year and promoted the adoption of a "Children's Code" by states and child welfare organizations. In Vermont the children in need of care under the new public welfare laws rapidly exceeded the ability of public and private agencies to provide the promised services. The meager Mothers' Aid allotments were quickly exhausted and proved insufficient to keep single mothers and their children out of poverty. Overseers of the poor had difficulty placing children in suitable foster homes, as local prejudices against their charges stood in the way. Referrals to the State School for the Feebleminded steadily mounted, as did the requests for placement in orphanages, usually restricted to children who were deemed healthy, normal, and emotionally stable.[36] Then, in the fall of 1918 the disastrous influenza epidemic struck. The "Spanish flu" proved more devastating to the Vermont population than the losses of soldiers fighting overseas. The population of the state in the 1920 census actually showed a decline since 1910, due to the mortality of war and disease combined. One-fourth of the deaths in 1918–1919 were caused by influenza; the young adult population was hit especially hard. Consequently, many children were orphaned, and resources for their care were overburdened.[37]

In November 1918 the Vermont Conference of Social Work responded to the disaster by appointing an Emergency Children's Aid Committee to collaborate with the American Red Cross in a statewide survey to locate children orphaned by the epidemic and assess their circumstances and needs. Sybil H. Pease, a professional social worker from the Boston regional office, was hired to conduct the study and act as executive secretary of the committee. Trained in social casework, which at that time involved careful scrutiny of the home environment of neglected and dependent children, Pease brought back bad news. Not only were local and state services inadequate to respond to the needs of orphans, but numerous other factors in rural Vermont had exacerbated the plight of children during the war and the epidemic. The other factors Pease found—desertion, tuberculosis, intemperance, and feeblemindedness—rekindled the "rural degeneracy" anxieties that Jeffrey, Dalton, and Flint had provoked. Sybil Pease's survey confirmed the consensus of Vermont social reformers, that the problems of Vermont children were serious and ubiquitous and that they demanded immediate action.[38]

Members of the Vermont Conference of Social Work held a special meeting in April 1919 to consider Pease's findings and decide what was to be done. As a result, they incorporated the Vermont Children's Aid Society, whose officers and about half its directors subsequently formed the advisory committee of the Eugenics Survey of Vermont. The mission statement of the Vermont Children's Aid Society makes no reference to eugenics or heredity, but the language of eugenics is pervasive. The purpose of the society, "to engage in child welfare work and social service designed to maintain the integrity of wholesome family groups," included cooperation with all agencies and officials involved in child and family welfare and carrying on "such work of prevention, relief, and remedy as will safeguard the welfare of minors and of the home." Relief and remedies might include family rehabilitation or finding suitable homes for dependent and neglected children. Two goals of the society, in particular, opened the door for eugenics: to study the "condition of dependent, neglected, and delinquent children" in Vermont and "to inform the public regarding conditions discovered."[39]

The Vermont Children's Aid Society, in collaboration with the Vermont Conference of Social Work, began immediately to develop formal connections with public and private institutions and to garner funds and expertise within Vermont and from out of state. They were united in their commitment to provide all the children in rural Vermont with the very best quality of social services available in the nation, services available only in large metropolitan areas in 1920. While the Children's Aid Society worked aggressively to expand foster care and adoption of needy children, they supported a number of other programs as well. They lobbied the state legislature for mental testing of delinquent and dependent children, regional psychiatric services, a complete census of all feebleminded Vermonters, and the standardization of child care to nurture *"the development of each child to the level of his potential capacity."* Leading experts from national organizations devoted to child welfare served as consultants.[40]

The Children's Aid Society hired experienced, professional social workers to apply their expertise in family and community casework to these newly discovered child welfare problems. Harriett E. Abbott and L. Josephine Webster were the first of these. Webster, a graduate of the Chicago School of Civics and Philanthropy, brought her experience as a social worker in the

Kentucky mountains, New York State, and the District of Columbia to her position as general secretary of the Children's Aid Society.[41] Harriett Abbott, a graduate of Vassar in 1895 and the Chicago School of Civics and Philanthropy in 1914, had been an investigator for children's aid societies in Illinois and New York before coming to Vermont. Both of these women would be connected with the Eugenics Survey of Vermont; Abbott would serve as field investigator for the first two years of its life.

Professional expertise was not necessarily appreciated in Vermont unless it had local roots or was supported by reputable Vermonters. The Vermont Children's Aid Society claimed to have selected its directors on the basis "of their humanitarian interests, standing and influence in their communities and geographical representation"—or perhaps of their well-developed missionary instincts. Perkins would follow the precedent; his advisory committee would include officers and directors of the Children's Aid Society who had been lauded by the *Burlington Free Press* as "some of the state's most prominent and philanthropic workers."[42] In fact, the Eugenics Survey would be funded by two of them. In a state famous for its respect for privacy, for minding one's own business, and for resenting intrusion into local affairs by state authorities or other "outsiders," the confidential information these social pioneers were able to gather is truly remarkable. The scope and influence of their efforts may be due in large measure to the fact that the leaders and advisors of such surveys were trusted Vermonters.

To expedite the exchange of information among officials and agencies engaged in social work, many states had a "central index" administered by the Department of Public Welfare to coordinate services to the social problem group. In 1920, Josephine Webster, general secretary of the Children's Aid Society, collaborated with the state Board of Charities and Probation to develop such an index. The "confidential" State Social Service Exchange promised to prevent conflicting treatment plans and relieve families of redundant "embarrassing investigations" by different agencies.[43] Perhaps unintentionally, the Social Service Exchange also created a broader visibility of problem families to social workers and others with access to the files. Initially, only the Children's Aid Society, the Burlington Red Cross, and city poormaster had used the files regularly, though many agencies throughout the state contributed their active cases to it. The information network no doubt improved the services to those families who wanted them. It also provided evidence of Vermont's unmet needs in family and child welfare, and the Legislative Committee of the Vermont Conference of Social Work used the information network in its crusade for legal reform.

One of the successful uses of the confidential case files was the reform of the marriage laws. L. Josephine Webster attributed the new legal age limit on marriage (fourteen for girls and sixteen for boys) to the convincing evidence from their case records of two dozen "little girl marriages *which were re-sulting disastrously to the social and economic welfare of the state.*" Parents of these "little girls" of age twelve, thirteen, and fourteen were blamed for arranging marriages to much older men in order to relieve them of their parental responsibility. Such unions, their files revealed, had ended in abandonment, abuse, destitution, mental illness, and frequently prostitution.[44]

Children's Aid Society workers Josephine Webster and Harriett Abbott were particularly concerned with the welfare of girls and young women. "The adolescent girl is our greatest problem," Webster explained in reference to the thirty-six unmarried mothers and infants they had served. While adolescence was a trying time in the best of circumstances, it was "a time of peril for girls hampered by poor heredity, lack of proper training, and often a personal experience of degradation and vice."[45] While Abbott and Webster helped "good mothers" secure jobs, Mothers' Aid, or child support from absent fathers, they also personally assisted in the rescues of a number of other young women from "unwholesome" home environments that promised a future of immorality and the ensuing social rejection, poverty, and decadence that they would, presumably, visit upon their own children. (See fig. 2.1.) Depending on age, circumstances, and available options, such girls might find themselves in suitable foster homes, the School for the Feebleminded in Brandon, the Colony for Feebleminded Women, or the Vermont Industrial School. Their names and the services rendered were added to the accumulating files of children with problems in families with problems.[46]

While state lawmakers responded favorably to the evidence concerning "little girl marriages," the Committee on Social Legislation of the Vermont Conference of Social Work, chaired by Asa Gifford (see fig. 2.2), failed to arouse support for two much-desired reforms. The first was the enactment of a state Children's Code, which would raise the standards of child care and define more specifically the conditions of neglect that demanded intervention. The second desired reform was a state census of feebleminded and mentally disturbed persons living outside institutions. "Vermont needs a mental survey which will locate every case of mental defect within our borders," Gifford argued in 1921, "and facilities for thorough psychiatric examination of all dependent and delinquent individuals." Such tests, Gifford insisted, would reveal the "intellectual grade or capacity . . . defects, tendencies, dispositions, and characteristics" that contributed to nearly all cases of chronic poverty and delinquency. Of particular concern was the "large class of Morons"—those not sufficiently handicapped to require institutionalization but who, without special training, would become the delinquents and the town charges of the future. Gifford pleaded on their behalf: "The call for thought and care comes from Morons in all parts of our commonwealth: 'Come and help us—for we can not help ourselves; and in helping us to avoid

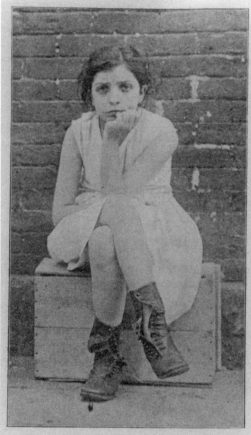

The maiden of today is the mother and home-builder of tomorrow. The treatment she receives today means weal or woe for many to come.

2.1 This illustration accompanied Harriett Abbott's report "True Stories of Vermont Children," a survey of child neglect cases resulting from negligent, immoral, and incompetent mothers.

First Annual Report of the Vermont Children's Aid Society, 1920.

Courtesy Vermont Children's Aid Society, Inc., Winooski, Vermont.

evil and error you will be serving your own interests and the welfare of your own children as well.'"[47] Unlike the plight of the child wives, the plight of the morons did not impress the state legislature sufficiently to fund a state census or mental testing program, despite the agitation on its behalf. Meanwhile, they multiplied on the Brandon waiting list, in the reform school, and in the confidential registry of people receiving or needing social services.

Despite the disappointing progress in some areas of state social services, the collaboration of the Children's Aid Society and the Department of Public Welfare gave the reformers a sense of control over the fate of dependent children in the state. Around 1920 pride in the progress made toward managing child welfare began to replace alarm over rural degeneracy, as the child

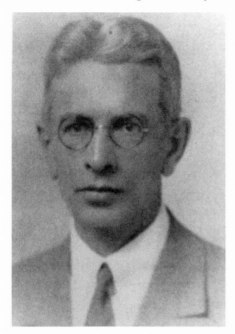

2.2 Professor Asa Gifford, president, Vermont Children's Aid Society, and chairman of the Committee on Social Legislation of the Vermont Conference of Social Work.

Henry Bergman and Vonda Bergman, "These Are Our Own: The Vermont Children's Aid Society Comes of Age," *The Vermonter: The State Magazine*, August 1940, p. 4.

rescuers discovered they were able to convert many hopeless and helpless families into self-supporting, responsible ones. Families that complied with remedial efforts and responded favorably to their social diagnosis and rehabilitation became the heroes in the new narratives of social reformers, which began to replace the tales of degeneracy after Children's Year. Willingness to work when a job was offered, the contribution of a portion of one's income to institutions that cared for their children, relinquishment of one's children to foster care or adoption if deemed necessary, or the transformation of a negligent mother into a nurturing one with the help of Mothers' Aid—all could shift many families from the category of pauper to "deserving" poor. Their stories served as testimonials to the ability of the new social reforms to "remedy conditions of evil" and to safeguard the family. The children were redeemed as well; in many of the narratives the imbeciles, cripples, and emotionally disturbed children were transformed by medical care and suitable foster homes into "perfectly normal" or "very bright" children with a promising future. Sometimes, children were removed from the corrupting influence of their parents and older siblings. W. H. Jeffrey presented stories like the following about John and Richard to illustrate the progress that had been made:

A few boards thrown together, one window, the floor for a bed, a stove, a table and three chairs comprised the home of John and Richard, and the rest of the family of seven—coming Vermonters, with the power of good or evil, growing up in a hovel. The father was sent to prison, the two older girls to Brandon, the mother placed in an institution, the apparently feeble-minded infant sent to the hospital where his throat, nose and ears were operated upon, and John and Richard were given necessary medical care. They are now bright, active boys who, if they have a chance will be an asset to Vermont, and the Board of Charities hopes to give them that chance.[48]

Other families remained in rebellion and sometimes hired lawyers to prevent child rescuers' attempts to repair the "broken little lives" of their children. They continued to be condemned to the class of "delinquent, dependent, and defective" Vermonters, and subsequently many of them came under the scrutiny of the Eugenics Survey. Transient or nomadic families presented a unique challenge to social workers. Not only was it difficult to assign responsibility for their care under Vermont's settlement laws, but their nomadic ways complicated the social worker's mission to diagnose their children's needs and cooperate with town officials to monitor the quality of parental care.

The Reorganization of State Government

The impulse to modernize, as reflected in human services and agriculture, was felt in state government as well. After World War I the national trends toward improving efficiency in government through centralization, the gradual shift of authority from the local to the state level, and the associated reliance of towns on state support precipitated a major restructuring of state government in Vermont. Government expenditures more than quadrupled in the first two decades of the twentieth century while the population increased by a modest 3 percent. Growing inequities among towns encouraged poorer towns to relinquish local authority and its associated costs to the state.[49] Vermont political leaders had struggled with this inequity since the turn of the century yet had jealously guarded the idea of town government as the true expression of direct democracy and Vermont self-sufficiency. Drawing once again on professional expertise from outside the state to assist with reforms in government administration, Vermont state leaders seriously began to consider ways to streamline operations and reduce costs. In 1917, at the request of Governor Horace F. Graham, the state Board of Control was established to centralize and consolidate the administration of finances, staffing of government offices, and coordination of state services.[50]

In 1918 the Board of Control hired consultants to conduct comprehensive reviews of the state administration and its management of state revenues.

Their report exposed a scrambled mess of overlapping authority, duplication and conflict of effort, waste of time and money, and lack of accountability at all levels. In response to these findings and to national trends in government reorganization, Vermont state services were completely reorganized. Seven departments were created to consolidate the diverse activities of the many boards, commissions, and supervisory committees that had proliferated in an ad hoc manner over the past fifty years. In this reorganization the Department of Public Welfare absorbed the duties and powers of all agencies and supervisory boards responsible for care of Vermont's "criminal, insane, feebleminded, wayward, and unfortunate (tuberculous, deaf, dumb, blind, poor) people."[51] For the first time in Vermont history, supervision and care of delinquents, the poor, and the handicapped was consolidated within a single state administrative entity.

The consolidation of public welfare services coincided with Asa Gifford's first legislative forum, where he presented a slate of recommendations for social legislation, drawn up by the Vermont Conference of Social Work's Legislative Committee, to convening state senators and representatives prior to the opening of the General Session. Because the commissioner of public welfare and many of his subordinates had advised Gifford's committee, his legislative forums offered the consensus of the state's professional experts and public officials on Vermont's particular welfare problems, their causes, and their remedies. Gifford's forums brought the "agitation and discussion" of the Vermont Conference of Social Work directly into the statehouse in an timely manner.

The Vermont state legislature could be a formidable obstacle to social reformers' efforts to enact the desired legislation to turn Vermont into a national model of rural child welfare services. L. Josephine Webster voiced the problem in 1920 in her address to the Vermont Conference of Social Work. "Vermont is unique," she argued. Its "well-known conservatism" and large, cumbersome legislature inhibited public improvements, requiring private agencies such as Webster's to assume responsibility and take the initiative for child helping that elsewhere was assumed by the state.[52] Because every town, large or small, had equal representation in the legislature, widespread public sentiment could facilitate legislative action where statehouse lobbying efforts failed. Unless a majority of lawmakers were convinced that a particular reform would appeal to their town leaders and neighbors or relieve local burdens rather than impose new responsibilities and expenses, they were unlikely to support it. Hence, raising public consciousness about the need for and value of more expensive welfare reforms was especially important.

There was one key legislative reform in the Vermont Conference of Social Work platform that had been implemented in many states but that the Vermont legislature refused to support: a state census of mentally deficient and psychologically disturbed Vermonters. Women who fell into these categories, every commentator agreed, were unequipped to provide the standards of child care demanded in a modern society. Apparently there were enough of them to cause concern, for their numbers were steadily growing in the central registry of Vermonters in need of special services or institutionalization. The Brandon State School for the Feebleminded, which was already overcrowded in 1920 and had a waiting list of fifty, needed expansion. Superintendent Truman Allen had convinced the state of the need to start a "colony" for "high-grade feebleminded women" in Rutland, but from his perspective, one colony was insufficient to deal with the problem. The collaboration of the Children's Aid Society and the state Board of Charities and Probation to find neglected children had expanded the caseloads of child welfare workers, as the courts, the Department of Public Welfare, and "desperate parents" responded to their offers of help. Children's Aid workers had difficulty finding suitable homes for about 20 percent of the children referred to them. Until the "apparent" mental defects in these infants and small children of "feebleminded parents" could be properly diagnosed as "real" or the "consequences of neglect," adoption of them was out of the question.[53]

Psychology professors at the University of Vermont had been promoting the use of psychometric testing in public schools and experimental problem child clinics for early detection of developmental disabilities. Children found to be mentally deficient or emotionally disturbed would then be eligible for special classes and services provided by trained psychiatric social workers. Mental testing of juvenile offenders, adult convicts, and recipients of poor relief, it was believed, should inform sentencing, rehabilitation and parole strategies, and placement in appropriate state institutions.

A state census of the mentally deficient and a comprehensive program of mental testing, however, would involve state expenditures, and without any evidence of need for such programs in Vermont, the conservative legislature would be unlikely to fund them. Perhaps in the interest of producing the necessary evidence, Harriett Abbott, district agent for the Children's Aid Society in Bellows Falls, Vermont, secured training in the summer of 1923 at the Eugenics Record Office in Cold Spring Harbor. She returned with the expertise to apply her skills and knowledge of Vermont families to locate relevant "defects" and also with the necessary training to turn her research into a public campaign for eugenic solutions.[54]

Eugenics as an Agent of Progressive Social Reform

While students in Professor Perkins's heredity class studied the army draft board results and learned about rural "cacogenic" families, social workers in the Children's Aid Society and the Department of Public Welfare continued to amass data on "unwholesome families" in need of social services. They began to notice that many new discoveries of child abuse or neglect, from "child wives" to unmarried mothers or recalcitrant parents who defied their warnings, were closely related to one another even though they had surfaced in different parts of the state. "Scarcely has a new case been brought to our attention," Josephine Webster observed, "that we do not know about it through some other work that has been done." Harriett Abbott's training at the Eugenics Record Office may have encouraged such discoveries, but the Social Service Exchange files facilitated them. As Webster explained, "past cases are a matter of record, not guess work." As new evidence accumulated on particular families, they began to assume a notoriety among welfare workers as incompetent parents, the source of neglected and "defective" children, and a growing "social cancer." The Children's Aid Society offered a variety of important services, including providing medical care for needy children, securing Mothers' Aid support or child support from wayward fathers, placing women and children in the State School for the Feebleminded, and issuing warnings or assisting the state's attorneys in prosecuting negligent parents. Yet Webster regarded the collection of information on the family conditions leading to child neglect as the most important function of her organization.[55] Meanwhile, in the Vermont Industrial School, Superintendent Charles Wilson and social worker Lena Hamilton collected the data on "family conditions" of two of their inmates from one of the "notorious, interrelated" families. They consolidated their findings on a pedigree chart displaying the incidence of mental defects, delinquency, and asocial tendencies of the family. This was certainly the chart that Perkins recognized as "a sort of Vermont Jukes picture."

In 1925, Perkins's vision for a eugenic study of Vermont converged with the interests of child welfare advocates when Mrs. Emily Proctor Eggleston provided Perkins with a $5,000 endowment to conduct a study of hereditary trends in the state. Mrs. Eggleston, a well-connected native Vermonter and an incorporator of the Vermont Children's Aid Society, paid the salary of Harriett Abbott, the first field-worker of the Eugenics Survey of Vermont, and provided transportation and office expenses. After its first year, Shirley Farr, a benefactor and director of the Vermont Children's Aid Society, continued the annual endowment until the survey closed in 1936. University of Vermont president Guy W. Bailey mediated these sponsorships; by mutual agreement, the source of the survey's funding was to be kept strictly confidential.[56]

Perkins adopted the "research and education" mission of the Vermont Children's Aid Society, but to their broader goal of "preserving wholesome family groups" he applied eugenics theory and methods. Following the precedent of the Vermont Conference of Social Work, Perkins defined the new organization as "nonsectarian and nonpolitical"—in other words, objective and aloof from special interests. Situating the Eugenics Survey in the university's Zoology Department evidently satisfied those requirements and affirmed the scientific nature of the enterprise. The new arrangement between private agencies and the Department of Public Welfare would make the construction of family pedigrees a relatively simple matter. Harriett Abbott would simply import information from the records of private agencies and state institutions and synthesize it into meaningful reports about Vermont's social problem group. A carefully selected advisory committee would ensure her access to the necessary files and grant her the authority to use the contents for dissemination of her findings.

Perkins's advisory committee, with its interlocking directorships in state government, academe, and charity work, secured the survey's position within Vermont's "progressive" coalition. The Vermont commissioners of public health, education, and public welfare and the superintendents of each of Vermont's correctional facilities and institutions for the insane and feebleminded represented the public sector. President Guy W. Bailey and psychology professor Asa Gifford of the University of Vermont and political science Professor K. R. B. Flint of Norwich represented the relevant fields in academe. L. Josephine Webster and Shirley Farr of the Vermont Children's Aid Society and Dr. Horace J. Ripley, superintendent of the Brattleboro Retreat, represented the interests of private charities. This alliance of public and private interest and of science, medicine, and social work represented a powerful synthesis of knowledge and authority, united in mission and vision.

Perkins's "nonsectarian and nonpolitical" advisory committee included no representatives of Vermont's working class or of ethnic minorities; their advocates were more often Roman Catholic priests or in some cases union leaders, who, of course, were excluded by definition. Nearly all persons involved in the survey were highly educated (most holding advanced degrees), Protestant (mostly Congregationalist), and affluent "Old American" stock, who shared a common allegiance to the celebrated virtues of Vermont's heritage. Perkins met with his advisory committee at least once a year. He sought its criticisms and suggestions and responded to them, and he advanced its social reform agendas in his publications. By acting as an agent for child welfare and social reform, Perkins was able to spread the gospel of eugenics beyond his classroom.

Some historians might find mental health and child welfare advocates' support for a eugenics survey in 1925 a little odd, if not downright unbelievable. Most histories of the mental health movement, social work, and child welfare reform suggest that by the mid-1920s eugenics had become anathema to enlightened psychologists and social workers; indeed their theories and therapies are said to have repudiated the idea of hereditary feeblemindedness. So why were Vermont's leading experts in all those fields supporting the Eugenics Survey of Vermont?

Certainly the members of the progressive coalition had not dispensed with heredity as a factor in many of the family problems that occupied their attention. While they might not have thought of the social problems of children in terms of "germplasm," they did think of them in terms of families. They were united in a belief in prevention strategies that targeted problems at their source. They were neither naive nor beguiled by Perkins's "expertise" in human genetics. They knew Perkins socially and professionally, as a Vermonter in good standing who was eager and willing to help them with their reform agenda. Most important, Perkins's survey promised to provide evidence they needed to secure support for the desired state services. Josephine Webster expressed the shared sentiment of the Children's Aid Society, certainly, when she announced, "We were glad to release a valued member of our staff, Miss Harriett E. Abbott, to work under the direction of the State University in making a eugenical study of Vermont. *No longer are child-caring agencies content to patch up broken little lives. Work of prevention is now recognized as even more important.*" Because child welfare agencies had procured such intimate knowledge of "the conditions that produced child neglect," Webster added, they felt accountable to "bring to the public not only the extent of this suffering but the underlying conditions which beget it."[57]

Social reformers' support for the Eugenics Survey also made sense in terms of where they stood on a particular learning curve: how to effect political change in Vermont. Since 1917 they had been frustrated with the failure of the largest state legislature in the smallest state in the union to offer social programs that more populous counties in other states (like Massachusetts) had in place. At the same time, they had discovered the power of their small, cohesive, and committed group of volunteers and civil servants to secure many reforms in social welfare, such as the marriage laws. Perkins's Eugenics Survey, if it produced enough evidence to persuade the legislature to support mental hygiene programs, could enlarge their influence within the small state. Hence, they willingly offered their reputations and expertise to promote progressive social legislation and its stepchild, eugenics.

While the Eugenics Survey promised to advance these political and professional agendas, it also satisfied, perhaps unconsciously, some psychological needs, not the least of which was to restore the state's reputation as a source of American talent, leadership, and character. Perhaps social reformers also stood to gain some sense of control over the family problems they had pursued and publicized, by projecting their own anxieties (over the future of their families and heritage) onto an unwitting and powerless "social problem group." From the perspective of the families and communities who became the objects of the search for "inherited defects," such a well-connected enterprise might well appear to be a conspiracy orchestrated by Vermont elites to "cleanse" the state of unwanted peoples. Certainly, deep historical prejudices emerged and were validated by the family studies. However, Perkins and his colleagues' belief in their own benevolence and their commitment to health and opportunities for children played important, if deceptive, roles. Unfortunately, the process of looking at people eugenically—in terms of their conformity to the idealized Vermont family—would alter the relationship between the middle class and the poor, between providers and recipients of "human services," and between the civil authorities and the people they served. In the public dissemination of their findings, the boundaries between fact finding and fault finding would dissolve, rendering members of the the social problem group more visible and more vulnerable to the broader fears and prejudices within Vermont communities. At the same time, their enterprise would become a struggle for the *meaning* of eugenics and a working out of its implications for Vermont.

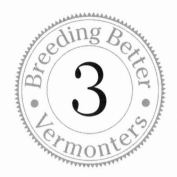

The Quest for a "Eugenic Vermont," 1925–1931

Eugenics means a deeper regard and satisfaction of our human nature. . . . Eugenics is the scientific projection of our sense of self preservation and our parental instincts.

—O. F. Cook, "Quenching Life on the Farm," 1928

The state is unique in the fact that 71 percent of the entire population is native to the State. No other state is as homogeneous as this. No other state, therefore, is challenged to the same extent to prove the quality of its native stock.

—Elin Anderson, *Selective Migration from Three Rural Vermont Towns*, 1931

In 1925, Henry Perkins had a very specific plan in mind: to turn the social records of families registered in the Vermont Children's Aid Society and the State Social Service Exchange into pedigrees of degeneracy that would help support a campaign for legalized sterilization. Recognizing that his success depended on securing the public trust and approval, Perkins relied heavily on his advisory committee for their advice and support in order to position the survey and himself, as director, as an advocate for Vermont communities, families, and children. Perkins's goal was to demonstrate the symbiosis of eugenics and Vermont traditions and, in the interest of social progress, convince his audience that eugenic solutions offered the best means "to make the waste places of the state bloom like the rose."

In 1925, Perkins and his supporters may have been unaware of another problem they would soon face: eugenics, as it had been conceived and applied thus far, was about to lose its appeal and scientific credibility. Between 1925 and 1931, because of that change, Perkins was forced to confront two challenges: he needed to adapt the rhetoric and ideas of eugenics to the agenda of his Vermont constituency and at the same time adapt his research and publicity to the changing climate of opinion among scientists and intellectuals regarding the merits of eugenics research and eugenic social policies.

Perkins addressed his first problem—that of creating public support for eugenics—by invoking familiar historical and cultural themes. The core ideology of eugenics—that a nation or race could fashion its own future through reproductive management—harmonized with the themes that were celebrated during Vermont's centennial years at the turn of the century: self-reliance, independence, and the state's unique role in American history. Vermonters were people who were born and bred in a rugged environment, in constant struggle against their neighbors' efforts to destroy their political autonomy, in order to create an independent republic. Perkins fused such Vermont historical legends with contemporary survey data to create a eugenic consciousness within a receptive Vermont audience and galvanize support for eugenics initiatives.

The Eugenics Survey of Vermont published five annual reports from 1927 to 1931 and also produced those included in *Rural Vermont: A Program for the Future*, the final report of the Vermont Commission on Country Life (VCCL, 1931). Together, these publications constitute the survey's public education mission and document how the meaning of eugenics in Vermont changed as Perkins sought its integration into the progressive reform agenda. The first six years of the survey can be divided into roughly three overlapping periods. During the early history of the survey, 1925–1928, Perkins publicized the survey's investigations of "degenerate" families in Vermont and launched a campaign for legalized sterilization. At the same time, he expanded eugenics research into a comprehensive statewide survey of all social forces that bore on the quality of the "Vermont stocks." In 1928–1929, Perkins adjusted eugenics research to the goals of the country life movement by turning "hereditary factors" into agents of progress or decline in rural communities and investigating social conditions that affected family size and quality. During the final period, 1929–1931, the Eugenics Survey, acting on behalf of the VCCL survey of "the Human Factor," studied the social forces affecting *population trends* within the state and their impact on the quality of rural town life and the maintenance of "desirable" families. In the country life context, members of the social problem group were redefined as handicapped persons, whose problems became the responsibility of the community, to be managed in cooperation with progressive social services.

"Early in the History of the Survey," 1925–1928

Perkins convened the advisory committee of the Eugenics Survey in September 1925 to discuss his "Proposal for a Good Eugenics Program" for Vermont and to authorize the research plan he had drafted. At this point his plan included all the unrealized goals of the Vermont Conference of Social Work: a census of the feebleminded, a program of mental testing of schoolchildren with state registration of all "defectives," the establishment of a state mental hygiene society, and an expansion of mental health and special education services to rural communities. With the exception of the sterilization law he included, Perkins's proposal resembled a program of mental hygiene more than it did the sort of eugenics program advocated by Charles Davenport and Harry Laughlin at the Eugenics Record Office in Cold Spring Harbor. His research plan included a survey of inmates of institutions, schoolchildren who were "retarded, backward, or behavior problems," recipients of poor relief, probation and parole cases, and other dependents served by private and public agencies. Perkins proposed to determine the distribution of "defectives" geographically (to see if there were "pockets of degeneracy" in particular rural areas), according to race (particularly French Canadians), and by family background. Perkins's proposed study of "notorious families," such as the ones already investigated by the Vermont Industrial School, would include genealogical study, casework on home conditions, characteristic social traits, and a survey of the families' representation in agencies of charity and corrections. Genealogical work would show cases of inbreeding and their consequences. The University of Vermont (UVM) Department of Commerce and Economics, he reported, had offered to assist the survey in its estimate of each family's expense to the state.[1]

Members of the advisory committee reacted favorably to Perkins's proposals and promised to assist Harriett Abbott with her study of the inmates of state institutions. Testing of schoolchildren was also a high priority for the advisory committee, because it would support a modified version of the "Massachusetts Plan" in Vermont, in which the Board of Education would be required to report all cases of backward and problem children to the Department of Welfare. They expected such a study to demonstrate the urgency of the desired expansion of facilities at the State School for the Feebleminded and colonies for the feebleminded. Perkins's advisors agreed to approach the

National Committee on Mental Hygiene (NCMH) for assistance in the mental testing of schoolchildren and in the organization of a Mental Hygiene Society in Vermont. Perkins predicted that Abbott's family casework would dovetail with the mental hygiene survey of schoolchildren, especially where children served by the Children's Aid Society belonged to "subnormal or dependent" families. Meanwhile the advisory committee would consider sterilization laws in other states. They agreed that the Eugenics Survey should "correlate all the material for perusal by the people of the state and for the state legislature." This plan was followed throughout the first three years of the survey.[2]

Perkins's fusion of eugenics with mental hygiene initiatives was timely, shrewd, and effective. New trends in social work in the 1920s drew largely on the developing field of psychology, and such research was heavily funded by the NCMH and associated philanthropies devoted to mental health. The mental hygiene advocates encouraged the establishment of child guidance clinics and had sponsored training and employment of "visiting teachers"; Perkins had included both programs in his eugenics plan. Visiting teachers assumed caseloads of emotionally disturbed or delinquent youths and became their advocates within the public school setting. Like specialists working with emotionally disturbed youth today, the visiting teachers helped their clients to adjust to the public school environment, and they also educated classroom teachers to respond to the emotional needs of disabled children rather than condemn their behavior. Mental and psychological testing instruments were elaborated within this context to provide a more scientific basis for the diagnosis of individual problems. Not surprisingly, social workers using the mental hygiene approach discovered that a considerable number of their clients were really suffering from emotional disorders or mental deficiency; social rejection precipitated various expressions of asocial behavior. Perkins, however, intended to prove that the family—via germplasm, social forces, or a combination of the two—was the root cause and vector of such disabilities and that restricting reproduction offered the best means of prevention.[3]

In October, Perkins described his plan for a "Survey of the Feebleminded in Vermont" at the annual meeting of the Vermont Conference of Social Work. Citing the draft board results and the preliminary genealogy work at the Vermont Industrial School as justification, Perkins explained that the survey on "interlocking families"—those connected by intermarriage and association with similar "families of a low order"—would shed light on Vermont's apparently high proportion of mental defectives. Perkins's address complemented Brandon State School superintendent Truman Allen's agitation for expansion of colonies for the feebleminded so that the congested facilities at Brandon could be used as a training school, not an asylum. The Conference of Social Work expressed its appreciation and approval for Perkins's survey in a formal resolution. Judge J. E. Weeks, commissioner of the State Department of Public Welfare and future governor, also commended the new survey as beginning "an important step in the program of the state of Vermont."[4]

Collecting Family Histories: Harriett E. Abbott

What the small eugenics society lacked in resources it made up for in the scope of its influence and the depth of its penetration into the family life and history of the social problem group. The energy and enthusiasm of Harriett E. Abbott, Perkins's first social worker, was in large measure responsible for the production of a large central file on Vermont's allegedly "dysgenic" families, whose members had found themselves as wards of the state or whose children had been classified as neglected by child helping agencies. In addition to twenty years of experience in child welfare, Abbott brought to the Eugenics Survey broad training in social research and related academic disciplines, the administration of public welfare, and the enactment of social legislation. As a graduate of the Chicago School of Civics and Philanthropy in 1914, Abbott's education in "scientific case work" had stressed "social diagnosis" for the purpose of recommending appropriate interventions for children, recipients of relief, and the delinquent population.[5] Her training at the Eugenics Record Office in Cold Spring Harbor in 1923 encouraged her to apply her skills in social diagnosis to eugenics field work—constructing pedigrees of families containing eugenically relevant information gathered from public agencies, charities, neighbors, and relatives. She would have been trained to trace alleged defects in pedigree charts to display their propagation through procreation. She was thereby sensitized to detect and diagnose evidence of feeblemindedness, insanity, and alcoholic, asocial, or criminal tendencies in designated families and to trace them back several generations.[6]

Harriett Abbott's assignment was to create a series of profiles of "defective" families, beginning with the information already on file with the Vermont Children's Aid Society and the Social Service Exchange. Her research then moved to the Vermont Industrial School and Brandon State School for the Feebleminded, where she gained additional information on particular inmates, many of whom owed their residency there to the child rescue efforts of the previous decade. She then surveyed the records of the inmates of Waterbury State Hospital for the Insane and the Vermont State Prison to locate parents, siblings, or other relatives of persons she found particularly interesting or promising. Her fieldwork consisted of visits to the hometowns of selected families to investigate home conditions, family size, and the mental status of any relatives to whom she had access. For the family histories, she consulted town clerks, records, overseers of the poor, and various "informants"—neighbors, teachers, ministers, and relatives willing to cooperate with the survey. For estimates of cost to the taxpayers, she queried town officials, Children's Aid Societies, and public institutions in Vermont and neighboring states. Abbott then constructed pedigree charts from her genealogical research, returning to institutional records to discover if relatives in "collateral branches" of these families were represented in state institutions.[7]

Families suitable for Abbott's eugenic investigations shared several characteristics: longevity in Vermont (several generations); neighbors, relatives, and acquaintances willing to share private family information with Abbott; and sufficient visibility in courts, poor relief records, and state institutions over time to demonstrate the continuity of "dependency, delinquency and defects" over successive generations. It is likely that some families targeted by the survey had been those who had defied interference of social workers and probation officers in their affairs in the past. Probably most were selected for study because they fit the stereotypical "cacogenic" families of rural America featured in the eugenics literature on which the Vermont survey was modeled. That the survey might be documenting histories of family exclusion, race and class prejudice, or even the consequences of long-standing disputes between neighbors and relatives did not seem to occur to Abbott, Perkins, or the influential supporters of the survey.

Harriett Abbott's field notes, investigative casework, and family profiles epitomize every aspect of eugenics work that mainstream opinion would find contemptible after 1930. Her language, assumptions, and reports were precisely the sort that would later identify eugenics as pseudoscience. Abbott was uninhibited in her negative value judgments of the families whose genealogies she constructed. She rarely hesitated in her positive diagnoses of feeblemindedness, mental incompetence, or the unsuitability for children of the home conditions she discovered. As the Eugenics Survey records are the only "confidential" case records in Vermont that have been made part of the public record, it is difficult to assess the extent to which Abbott's approach was typical of social workers of her period and training. Abbott's field notes and family histories document the same conditions and "defects" that had infuriated social reformers since 1915. Her case histories recorded alcoholism, sex offenses, allegations of or convictions for child neglect or domestic abuse, large age differences between husband and wife, and unsanitary living conditions—all previously featured in Vermont Conference of Social Work and Children's Aid Society annual reports. To these social diagnoses, Abbott added medical conditions like goiter and arteriosclerosis and tuberculosis to her summaries of each family. Abbott evidently consulted another source in the Eugenics Survey library, for nearly every medical and social condition she noted as "defects" can be found in the chapter titled "Who Should and Should

Not Marry" in *Woman: Her Sex and Love Life*, a contemporary marriage and sex manual by urologist Dr. William J. Robinson.[8]

The two features that place her research within traditional eugenics were genealogy and cost estimates of the "burden to the taxpayer" of selected families. Pedigree charts graphically documented cases of incest and cousin marriages, common law and multiple marriages, and intermarriage among other "notorious" families. Such revelations reinforced the belief that the source of Vermont's welfare problems lay within "unwholesome" families and suggested that heredity played a more crucial role than environmental deprivation. The genealogical study also expanded dramatically the number of persons whose private lives were scrutinized by social workers and public welfare authorities. While Eugenics Survey policy dictated strict confidentiality of all case records and protection of the identity of families and individuals studied from the general public, welfare workers and other "authorized investigators" were encouraged to consult the files as an extension of the State Social Service Exchange. At the end of the first year, Abbott had collected data on fifty families and over 3,500 individuals, encompassing several generations. Of these, ten families were selected for more extensive study over the following year. When the family studies were concluded in 1928, the Eugenics Survey had registered over six thousand individuals and had charted and developed family histories on sixty-two family lines (see Appendix B).

While Abbott conducted the research and prepared reports, Harry Perkins publicized her work and findings and collected materials for the Eugenics Survey library on all matters relating to eugenics, mental hygiene, and social work as references for eugenics research and interpretation. He also enlisted the support of the NCMH for a survey of mental and emotional deficiency among Vermont schoolchildren and lectured publicly to receptive audiences on eugenics and his survey's work. There is no evidence to suggest that he participated directly in the research or was acquainted with any of the families except by reputation. Virtually all data collection and compilation on Vermont families was performed by Abbott, her successors, and the survey's secretary, Anna Rome. By his own admission, Perkins's only training in eugenics had been from the professional literature, textbooks, and consultation with experts in the field, such as Charles Davenport at the Eugenics Record Office.[9] Yet he confidently asserted that the social problems of the state were based on heredity, which in turn placed tremendous economic burdens on the citizens of the state. In his new public role of eugenicist, progressive social reformers welcomed him into their inner circle. The Vermont Conference of Social Work elected him to their executive committee in 1926 and made him the program chairman for their next annual conference in Burlington. Perkins's report at their 1926 annual meeting on the progress of the survey's "census of the feebleminded" inspired Shirley Farr of the Vermont Children's Aid Society to fund the Eugenics Survey for the following year.[10]

Organizing for Therapeutic Intervention

In October 1926, Perkins convened the Eugenics Survey advisory committee for two specific purposes: to plan a campaign for legalized sterilization in the upcoming session of the state legislature of Vermont and to approve the NCMH's proposed survey of Vermont schoolchildren and special education services. The advisory committee approved the proposed alliance with the NCMH and turned toward a consideration of the sterilization issue, having read Harry Laughlin's pamphlet "Eugenical Sterilization to 1926," which Perkins had sent to them prior to the meeting. In light of the 1913 failure of a sterilization law in Vermont, Perkins proposed that a new bill should emphasize sterilization by consent, as in California. Dr. Truman Allen of the Brandon state school and Norwich University professor K. R. B. Flint, who had suggested sterilization of the feebleminded in *Poor Relief in Vermont*, both noted that sterilization was too frequently regarded as a replacement for institutions and colonies; the public should understand that sterilization was only one tool to assist in a mental hygiene program in the state. Dr. Allen noted that a law permitting sterilization would facilitate the discharge and parole of many of his charges at Brandon and thereby enable him to focus on the needs of more serious cases. The advisory committee agreed to promote a sterilization law and to study the laws in Maine, New Hampshire, Wisconsin, and California to draft a suitable bill. Perkins was directed, on Professor Flint's recommendation, to distribute copies of the American Eugenics Society's pamphlet, *A Eugenics Catechism*, to state legislators while Asa Gifford, as chairman of the Vermont Conference of Social Work's Committee on Social Legislation, incorporated a sterilization bill into the platform presented to the General Assembly in January 1927.[11]

Gifford's proposal for a sterilization law fell within the compass of his broad vision of social enrichment that would promote community cooperation, wholesome family life, and child welfare. Among classic progressive reforms calling for expanded Mothers' Aid, workmen's and widows' compensation for injuries or death of employees, and safeguards of minors, he also called for extended oversight and more rigorous documentation by the state in marriage and divorce proceedings, child custody and adoption, and the delivery of poor relief in towns. In regard to sterilization, he attempted to find common ground between private rights and the public interest: "*Sterilization* of Defectives, and of Chronic Delinquents and of certain Psychopathic Types. Permissive legislation should be enacted enabling the legal performance of an operation to sterilize where public policy requires and the individual (or in case of an incompetent, the guardian) consents thereto. The prevention of procreation by certain defective and deranged individuals would be an immense gain, social, moral, and economic."[12] The bill, "An Act Relating to Voluntary Eugenical Sterilization," was introduced in the state senate in February, the month following the publication of Perkins's first annual report, *Lessons from a Eugenical Survey of Vermont*, and his agreement to chair a state committee of the American Eugenics Society to promote sterilization.[13] While the progressive coalition introduced the surgical solution, Perkins's first annual report attempted to provide the substantive support.

Public Education on Vermont's Eugenics Problem

Perkins's first official publication of the Eugenics Survey, *Lessons from a Eugenical Survey of Vermont*, targeted a local audience consisting of two overlapping groups: the "sons and daughters of Vermont," who shared his allegiance to the state and his appreciation for blood lines and breeding, and civic leaders and officials who were struggling to administer the public relief and child welfare laws. For the latter group, the options were running out as the available institutions were already overcrowded, and "dependent and neglected" children were no longer permitted in poorhouses or poor farms. Perkins taught the eugenic lessons by translating local legends into classic rural eugenics narratives. Despite his assertions that the Eugenics Survey was a purely scientific, fact-finding enterprise, he made his appeal to longstanding local prejudices. He amplified the tension between town pride and frustration in meeting their obligations to the poor and offered eugenic sterilization and mental hygiene programs as solutions.

Perkins modeled the survey's report of its preliminary findings on the narratives of Arthur E. Estabrook, who had first popularized eugenic explanations for rural "pockets of degeneracy" in his studies *The Jukes in 1915* and *The Nam Family: A Study in Cacogenics*. Estabrook's standard themes were isolation and inbreeding, unconventional sex and family relationships, and, when applicable, miscegenation among White settlers, Indians, and sometimes "Negroes." He then associated these patterns, through the construction of genealogy and pedigrees, with delinquency, child neglect, and illiteracy and public expense, obtained through public records. Each field study was a variation of these themes. In his 1926 study, *Mongrel Virginians: The Win Tribe*, for example, Estabrook profiled a triracial group of families of five hundred members living in an isolated region of the Blue Ridge Mountains. The Win Tribe, he judged, originated from the social rejects of Native American, White, and African American communities, who then concentrated their alleged innate inferiority through interbreeding and incorporating additional members like themselves each generation. This study may have appealed to Perkins, since Abbott had selected some multiracial families for intensive investigation.

More likely, Estabrook's study "The Tribe of Ishmael" (1920) may have provided Perkins with the eugenic profile for his story of the Vermont "Gypsy Family." Estabrook's "Ishmaelites" were concentrated in the state of Indiana and had been made notorious in the late nineteenth century by a minister in the National Conference of Charities and Corrections who had studied and publicized their frequent appearances in penitentiaries, almshouses, and charity lists. When Estabrook expanded the genealogies of the Ishmaels, he concluded that in 1885 the tribe comprised about six thousand, stemming from four hundred different family heads whose descendants were distributed throughout the midwestern states. He traced the "central family" to "John Ishmael," whose ancestors left the Kentucky mountains in 1790, and his "half-breed" wife, who started the Indianapolis clan around 1825. Their descendants had intermarried with other nomadic families whose ancestors, Estabrook suggested, were some of the "criminals, paupers, and prostitutes" deported to the colonies from England in the seventeenth and eighteenth centuries. All of these theoretically related families were noted for the "outstanding characteristics" of "pauperism, licentiousness, and gypsying."[14]

Estabrook referred to the Ishmaelites as the "American gypsies." He theorized that John Ishmael, the founder of the family, had started the tradition of wandering during summer months into the Indian reservations of the Midwest, living off the land by hunting and fishing and returning in the fall to "civilization" in Indianapolis. There they would winter over in poor asylums or "get their names on the trustee's books before the frost appeared." Over the decades, as the Indians were being pushed from their reservations and White settlements spread across the frontier, the American gypsies had to wander farther west, sometimes remaining away over the winter, presumably in a county poorhouse in another state. As land settlement expanded, Estabrook explained, the Ishmaelites found it increasingly difficult to live off the countryside and resorted to begging and stealing when necessary. Families would band together in wagon parties, "swapping horses, gambling, and living as best they might." The American gypsy culture, Estabrook argued, created the opportunity for mating among similar types, thereby concentrating and spreading "the antisocial traits of their germplasm" throughout the whole Middle West.[15]

Estabrook's story of the "Tribe of Ishmael" reads more like a parable than a report of scientific or historical research. He appropriated nearly every metaphor and pathology that would invoke anxiety or revulsion in his audience: the idea of racial mixing, the incest taboo, sexual licentiousness, safety of personal property, and ambivalence over the giving and receiving of charity. By virtue of their transience, their disregard for legal boundaries between American settlers and native peoples, and their way of life beyond the moral, social, and geographical boundaries of American civilization, the American Gypsies represented the antithesis of respectable middle-class values. Interestingly, Perkins did not publicly mention the Ishmaelites as he had Estabrook's other families. He simply superimposed the Ishmael fable on one very old kinship network in Vermont.

The "Gypsy family" of Vermont was one of the first and most extensively studied kinship networks in the survey. Harriett Abbott's genealogical work had traced the family line back five generations to an ancestor from Quebec of "mixed ancestry with apparently very strong doses of Indian and Negro." His descendants, Perkins claimed, retained "their ancestor's roving or Gypsy tendency. . . . They are horse traders, fortune tellers, and basket makers." Like the Ishmaelites, Perkins's Gypsies wintered over in "rural settlements not far from the city" and spent summers in roving wagon bands helping themselves to the personal property of residents in rural communities, selling baskets, trading horses, and telling fortunes. Like the Ishmael phenomenon in the Midwest, Perkins's Vermont Gypsies had "contributed liberally to the population of prisons and other institutions of Vermont, New York, and Massachusetts." What was startling about the Gypsy family is that, over a period of four months, Abbott had been able to triple the number of descendants and relatives of these families, bringing their numbers to 436. Not only were Abbott's sources providing information liberally to the survey, the so-called Gypsies also had large families.[16]

Perkins pointed out that "they are not real gypsies. . . . Their only claim to the term 'gypsy' is their dark skin." Moreover, Abbott's genealogical research had traced their origins to early-nineteenth-century immigrants from Quebec. For Perkins's audience, these families occupied an obvious place in the Vermont visions of the past. They bore a resemblance to the "inferior class" of French Canadians that Rowland E. Robinson claimed had "infested the state" and then mysteriously disappeared, but they also seemed a lot like the Native American nomadic families that nineteenth-century Vermonters had also called Gypsies.[17] In fact, recent research by the Abenaki people has revealed that Perkins and Abbott's Gypsy family were indeed Abenaki families who had maintained their native ways to the extent that they were able in New England. The survey's portrayal of the Gypsies as primitive, illiterate, and "looked upon with wholesome fear by the people who know them" no doubt massaged historic, latent prejudices against the people who sold baskets, miniature canoes, and other Indian crafts to support themselves and sustain their culture. Perkins's emphasis on their transience supported, perhaps inspired, Asa Gifford's legislative reform requiring registration of all dependent and neglected children "whose parents are Vermont rovers or nomads with no legal settlement" as wards of the state.[18]

Perkins featured two other examples of Vermont "degeneracy" in his *Lessons*: the Pirates and the Chorea Family. Both of these groups were well known in Vermont and in Burlington in particular. Huntington's chorea was one of the genetic conditions Charles Davenport attributed to a dominant gene (a theory that endures in the present). A considerable medical literature existed on this disease, its diagnosis, its various manifestations, and its incidence. The Vermont family diagnosed with Huntington's chorea was already known to Charles Davenport and Henry Goddard at the Vineland Training School in New Jersey, where some of its members had been patients. The State Hospital for the Insane at Waterbury included patients diagnosed (correctly or not) with Huntington's chorea, and on visiting days the public could go and see patients afflicted with chorea and other mental illnesses. Perkins simply drew on the eugenics and genetic research to educate the Vermont lay public on chorea's genetic origin, its incidence in Vermont, the suffering it caused affected individuals and their families, and the public expense required for care and treatment. Perkins predicted that the disease would die out, as the afflicted families appeared to be having fewer children.[19]

The Pirate family, however, had no real counterpart in the broader eugenics literature but was very well known locally. The Pirates, really an extended lake-dwelling family, had lived for generations in houseboats, earning their living by transporting goods up and down Lake Champlain. During winter months they docked in the Burlington harbor and other ports on the Vermont and New York side of Lake Champlain. Like the American Gypsies, they lived close to but not within the conventional boundaries of American culture. Since Harry Perkins's childhood, these families had been scorned by Burlington's civic-minded elites. After the turn of the century, intolerance mounted as the houseboat culture became increasingly viewed as detrimental to the interests of owners of lakeshore properties. Perkins's generation nicknamed them Pirates; they were frequently accused of theft, extortion, and "loose living," and their houseboats and shanties near the lake shore were portrayed as breeding grounds for disease.[20] Perkins's eugenics lesson on the Pirates portrayed them as a threat to public health and safety. They lived "in utmost squalor and destitution. . . . Disease and feeblemindedness are always conspicuous in the children." They were "the terror" of property owners and boat owners because of their "thieving habits" and were suspected of turning a profit on the food and clothing they received from sympathetic, charitable people. Moreover, Perkins's Pirates were elusive and out of control: "As soon as things get too hot for them in one locality they pull up stakes and move to the next town or port. . . . They manage pretty successfully to keep out of prison, although frequently arrested for petty larceny and various other minor offenses."[21]

The story of how these families became interesting to the social work establishment and the further intrusion in their family life in the wake of Abbott's genealogical research lies beyond the scope of this study and belongs to the families involved. Harriett Abbott apparently found it easy to obtain information on these families, an unlikely achievement without cooperation among those who knew them. Once registered within the public welfare and social agency network, the ultimate effect on these families must have been considerable.

Perkins emphasized Harriett Abbott's "tactful detective work," the fact-driven nature of the enterprise, and its endorsement by local and national organizations devoted to social betterment, but his litany on the Pirates, the Gypsies, and the Chorea Family was less a scientific report than a sermon on eugenics, designed to illustrate his "one great lesson": The difference between wholesome and antisocial families was not rooted in problems of the will, the spirit, or the lack of sound Christian upbringing, as social reformers had argued in the past. It was rooted in deep biological differences and "hard heredity": "Without making too positive an assertion, I think we can safely say that in the sixty-two families that we have studied at any rate, 'blood has told,' and there is every reason to believe that it will *keep right on* 'telling' in future generations. 'Running water purifies itself.' The stream of germplasm does not seem to."[22]

Perkins intimated that the survey's preliminary findings on such families were a conservative estimate of the problem of degeneracy throughout Vermont rural communities, which would only worsen because the families involved were prolific and their children grew up amid immorality and destitution. Abbott's investigations had revealed a flagrant disregard for enforcement of marriage and divorce laws. "Common law marriages are all too common," Perkins noted, and Abbott's failure to obtain information indicated an inexcusable laxness on the part of local officials to maintain vital records.

The remainder of Perkins's report outlined the main thrusts of the mental hygiene initiatives supported by the Eugenics Survey and the social legislation Gifford had introduced the same month. In discussing sterilization, Perkins pointed out that twenty-three states had laws for compulsory sterilization of mentally defective persons for eugenic purposes (not punishment). Citing the California studies, Perkins mentioned that half of the sterilizations were "voluntary," that is, performed at patients' request or consent, when they had come to understand their condition was hereditary and that "the treatment" would enable them to once again live freely in society. Eugenic sterilization would apply only to those whose defects were clearly inherited and would complement special education and psychiatric clinics for problem children.

Perkins concluded the report with a discussion of the "rights of the individual," meaning those "decent citizens" whose freedom and safety were compromised by the growing burden and threat of "lawless, immoral, degenerate, and mentally defective" persons living and breeding in their midst. Perkins's message was this: bad germplasm not only compromised the tenuous prosperity of rural communities, but it threatened the security, liberty, and pursuit of happiness of deserving citizens and their children.[23]

Despite the efforts of Perkins and his colleagues on behalf of sterilization, the bill passed by the state senate on March 15, "An Act Relating to Voluntary Eugenical Sterilization," was immediately and soundly defeated in the house in a vote of 126 to 54 two days later. Perkins later attributed its failure to overzealousness on the part of some proponents who had unintentionally prejudiced the case. A year later, Asa Gifford noted that the chief obstacles to improved social legislation in general were the "unenlightened state of public opinion regarding the problems involved" and "the presence of reactionary politicians in strategic places on committees of the Legislature."[24] The attempt at a sterilization law may have been premature, however. Two months after its defeat, the U.S. Supreme Court upheld Virginia's eugenic sterilization law in the famous case *Buck v. Bell*, in which Oliver Wendell Holmes's opinion that sterilization of mentally deficient persons, like vaccinations for smallpox, fell within the police powers of the states. This decision reinvigorated campaigns for sterilization throughout the nation.[25]

Perkins may have realized that a more thoughtful public education campaign was needed, rather than the appeal to the popular prejudices that his "lessons" on the Gypsies and Pirates had offered. After the first annual report, Perkins dropped all references to Pirates and Gypsies. Conceivably some of Perkins's constituency found these stereotypes offensive, uncharitable, and in poor taste. Perhaps the real or imagined presence of such families in Vermont was detrimental to the image of the state that the tourist board was so actively promoting in those years. Because families categorized as Pirates and Gypsies had French Canadian ancestry, they may have sought refuge in the Catholic Church from assaults on their character and social workers' intervention in their private lives. The numbers alone suggest quite another problem, however. The kinship groups in Abbott's records were long established in Vermont and had at one time been integral, if marginalized, members of Vermont communities. As the genealogies of these and other "degenerate" families expanded, Perkins and his colleagues discovered many highly respected and well-connected relatives in the pedigrees—the very respectable Vermonters whose interests Perkins had claimed to protect. Truman Allen had warned Perkins in 1926 of offending Vermonters through the categorical condemnation of the feebleminded and insane as accidents of bad breeding.[26] Perhaps he had gone too far.

That summer, Perkins pushed forward the completion of the family studies, the statistical compilations of their findings, cross-referencing and indexing, and the estimates of taxpayers' expenses—for town and private charity,
court costs, and incarceration or institutionalization—for ten of the families.
He hired two more social workers to assist Abbott and Rome in the effort.
Francis Conklin, also a trainee at the Eugenics Record Office, provided particular expertise in statistics for the final reports. Conklin would replace Abbott after Abbott left the survey in September 1927 for further training in
psychiatric social work. The NCMH survey of mental deficiency in schoolchildren was underway, and Perkins no doubt wanted the results of the family
studies to complement their findings so that he could present them to the
Vermont Conference of Social Work at their October annual meeting. Moreover, Perkins wanted to bring the first phase of eugenics study to an end in
order to broaden the scope of the Eugenics Survey.

The Comprehensive Rural Survey

Early in 1927, Perkins renewed his request for a sabbatical to organize a comprehensive study of rural Vermont. Perkins wanted to survey *all* factors—social, economic, cultural, and hereditary—that were contributing to the rural
exodus and decline in the quality of life in many towns. Such a comprehensive study, he hoped, would reveal the relationships between human heredity
and environmental influences and the nature of their interaction. At this
point, Perkins admitted that his social workers had become convinced that
problems of delinquency and deficiency in Vermont were affected and perhaps caused by rural conditions. Perkins found support for his plan among
members of the Eugenics Survey advisory committee and various national
organizations that funded such projects. UVM President Guy W. Bailey
granted Perkins a sabbatical for the 1927–1928 academic year to organize the
project.[27]

Perkins's sabbatical year was a period of trial and error as he attempted
to expand the Eugenics Survey's mission beyond the confines of traditional
eugenics family work. The comprehensive survey would require additional
investigators, more funding, wider participation, and the cooperation of local
organizations and state agencies with an interest in rural improvement.
Perkins pushed forward parts of the eugenics agenda and retreated from others. He elaborated, adapted, and refined the survey's mission to appeal to
Vermonters' concerns, to attract funding from major granting agencies, and
to enhance the scientific credibility of his enterprise.

Perkins's planning of the Vermont Conference of Social Work 1927 annual
meeting is one example of the inherent difficulty of incorporating eugenics

into a program of social improvement. To promote the theme, "Rural Better-ment in Vermont," Perkins had invited speakers and organized round-table discussions to promote positive developments in education and medical care and the establishment of "community houses" as social centers in rural towns. But Perkins also had invited two national leaders in American eugenics to address the convention: Leon Whitney, executive director of the American Eugenics Society, and Judge Harry Olson, chief justice of the municipal court of Chicago and commissioner of the International Congress of Eugenics. Both of these ardent eugenicists strongly urged their Vermont audience to mount an aggressive campaign to prevent the reproduction of the unfit in order to guard the future of the race. The negative approach may not have played well to this audience in this particular context. On the recommenda-tion of his advisory committee, Perkins directed Francis Conklin to take the opposite approach: to study the "better branches" of the families previously stigmatized as degenerate by the Eugenics Survey. The better branches would serve as the control group for their deficient relatives (whose numbers had multiplied dramatically in the family pedigrees over the summer) and present Vermont family life in a more positive light. If the leaders of the Ver-mont Conference of Social Work were offended by Perkins's promotion of negative eugenics, they forgave him for it, for they congratulated him on his efforts at the Burlington meeting and elected him president for the follow-ing year.[28]

Conclusion of the Search for Vermont Degeneracy: The "Doolittles"

While Conklin surveyed the better branches of one of the ten special pedi-grees and continued statistical work on the family data, Perkins wrestled with two serious dilemmas as he prepared the Eugenics Survey's second annual report. The NCMH had completed its survey of schoolchildren and had re-ported that Vermont's rate of mental deficiency was comparable to the na-tional average, in contrast to the army draft board results that Perkins had used to justify the survey's pedigree work in 1926. The NCMH team had re-leased only statistical summaries of their findings and recommendations for improved mental hygiene services. Furthermore, their failure to provide the identity of children found mentally deficient foiled Perkins's plan to conduct pedigree work on their families. Having promised the results of this study in his first annual report, Perkins now faced the challenge of demonstrating the importance of his eugenics research when it appeared that Vermont had a *normal* incidence of mental deficiency.

Perkins's second problem was his public agitation for eugenic sterilization the previous spring. Not only had his efforts failed, but his exploitation of the survey's findings to promote a politically and religiously controversial bill had compromised the purely scientific motivation he had claimed for his enterprise. On the national scene, American eugenicists were now being openly criticized by intellectual leaders and by some biologists for their exploitation of genetics for political ends, the transparent race and class prejudices in most of the work, and their diversion of research time and money from experimental work on genetics to poorly conceived studies on social conditions, whose causes were more likely environmental. After the developments of 1927, Perkins knew his credibility as a scientific, impartial arbiter of human issues was in jeopardy.[29]

Perkins used his second annual report (March 1928) to conclude the first phase of the Eugenics Survey's work and announce its new role as investigator of rural conditions. Perkins backed off his previous promotion of sterilization by emphasizing the survey's role in general *research* into the sources and causes of social problems in Vermont—research that *"can be used for social betterment in Vermont*—that is, for the ultimate improvement of the quality of our citizens."[30] Because the Eugenics Survey advisory committee had favored the sterilization law in 1927, Perkins explained, many Vermonters labored under the misconception that such legislation constituted their *whole* purpose. Perkins reviewed the broader goals and activities of the survey, including its intimate involvement with the Vermont Conference of Social Work, its new study of better branches of degenerate families, its collaboration with the NCMH, and its assistance during the flood of 1927. The survey's most important project, Perkins announced, would be a comprehensive survey of all rural conditions that influenced the quality of family life in Vermont. "The Eugenics Survey is not only the initiator of this plan but will be its center and core if it is carried out," Perkins predicted.[31]

Despite Perkins's attempts to qualify the survey's position on sterilization and to promote the positive face of eugenics, the second annual report featured one of the Harriett Abbott's "finished studies," leaving little doubt about the focus, nature, and purpose of the first three years of eugenics work or their continued support for negative eugenics measures. Perkins selected for publication one of Abbott's final reports on one of the first families surveyed: "The Results of the Matrimonial Adventures of Four Degenerate Offspring of the Fourth Generation of the Dumston Family." For the annual report the pseudonym "Doolittle" was substituted for Dumston, and the title was shortened to "An Expensive Luxury," adding ridicule to the humiliation of being investigated in the first place. The report surveyed the complete spectrum of Vermont problems of dependency and delinquency. It revealed the effectiveness of the survey in obtaining highly specific and confidential information on Vermonters and displayed the data in a manner that few, if any, Vermonters had ever seen before.

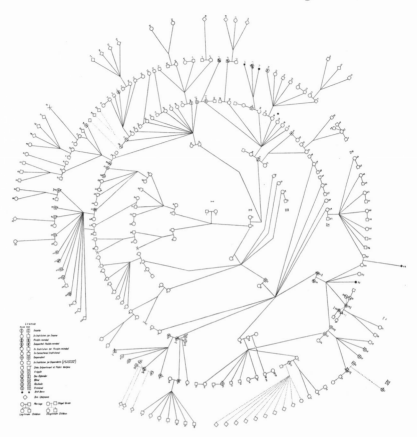

3.1 Clock-dial chart of the "Doolittle" family. (Enlarged detail on page 89.) *Second Annual Report of the Eugenics Survey of Vermont*, 1928. Courtesy Special Collections Department, University of Vermont Library.

Perkins displayed the family's pathologies and misfortunes on a fold-out "clock dial" pedigree chart, like the ones in other eugenics publications.[32] This interesting modification of a standard pedigree chart was intended to condense the unwieldy pedigrees of families studied onto a single page. It also gave the unmistakable image of a spreading and growing social cancer, or epidemic of immorality, crime, and incompetence, stemming from a single couple and propagated through sexual reproduction. The radiating circles of "defects" and their astonishing multiplication, accumulation, and concentration in recent generations resembled a rupturing abscess, which had festered for generations through multiple cousin and common law marriages, illicit unions, unbridled sexuality, and excessive fecundity. (See fig. 3.1.)

Abbott's descriptions of the Doolittles was vague about the exact nature of

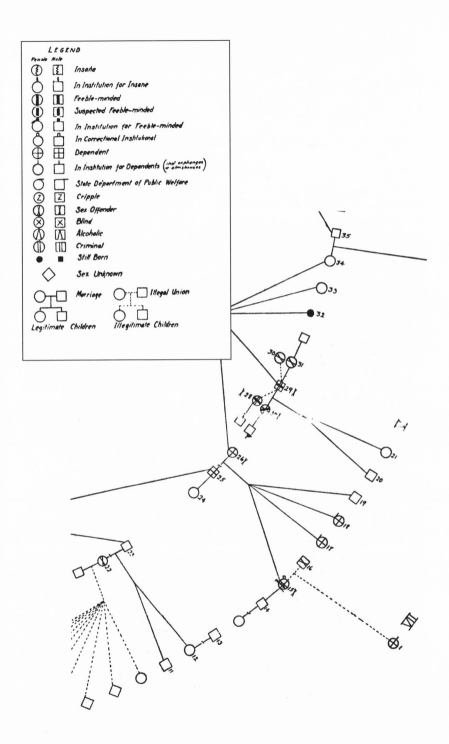

LEGEND

Female	Male	
⊘	⊡	Insane
○	⬓	In Institution for Insane
◑	⊞	Feeble-minded
◐	⊟	Suspected Feeble-minded
○	⬚	In Institution for Feeble-minded
○	⬚	In Correctional Institutional
⊕	⊞	Dependent
○	⬚	In Institution for Dependents (incl orphanges or almshouses)
○	⬚	State Department of Public Welfare
Ⓩ	☒	Cripple
⊘	⬚	Sex Offender
⊗	☒	Blind
◉	⬚	Alcoholic
◍	⊞	Criminal
●	■	Still Born
◇		Sex Unknown

○—□ Marriage   ○┈□ Illegal Union

○—□   ○┈□
Legitimate Children   Illegitimate Children

their condition or circumstances ("immoral, feebleminded, and inadequate") and most precise and uncompromising regarding the unfitness for parenthood of some of the Doolittles. Her diagnoses were based largely on court and poor relief records or the type of institution in which parents and children were found, suggesting that some of the "degenerate" families owed this investigation to an earlier breakup of "unwholesome" families after Children's Year. Sterilization was never mentioned but certainly was implied in Abbott's suggestion that "the state of Vermont would have been better off had Richard, Simon, John, and Joseph of Generation III not been allowed to produce children."[33] She qualified her argument, stating that the data also showed cases in which high-quality homes had made several of the Doolittles' offspring into respectable citizens.

While Perkins and Abbott equivocated on whether the cause of the "social and economic drag" of the Doolittles was genetic or social, their estimates of the public expenses for the misfortunes of the family would have exacted little sympathy from the respectable middle class. Not only had this family cost the states of New York, New Hampshire, and Vermont over $15,000 annually in relief and institutional care, but they habitually crossed state boundaries, eluded the efforts of social and public agencies to find them, and often left handicapped and neglected children in their wake. The Doolittle case also provided an opportunity for dovetailing eugenics with mental hygiene, which Perkins had promised in 1925. Throughout her report, Abbott argued for every mental hygiene initiative the progressive coalition had supported— child guidance clinics, early diagnosis of mental deficiency through intelligence testing, and special education classes. Such programs promised to reduce the drain on public revenues resulting from the delinquency and dependency of persons like the Doolittles.[34]

Abbott's field notes and correspondence demonstrate the uninhibited flow of information on individuals within the social rehabilitation network. In the case of "Maggie Simpson," one young woman in the Doolittle clan, for example, Abbott's detailed report reveals her relentless pursuit of information and her particular concern with attractive, sexually active young women who flaunted the conventions of middle-class society. It is impossible to determine from the records what had actually gone wrong with Maggie Simpson. Had she suffered a mental breakdown from a stressful life, had she defied the efforts of authorities to rehabilitate her, or was she really as disabled as Abbott claimed? Maggie had been a ward of the state as a child. She had been placed in an orphanage and, failing to make the expected adjustment there, had spent her adolescent years in psychiatric hospitals and the Vermont Industrial School. She was then "set free" by a sympathetic judge who had responded to her pleas not to be recommitted, despite her IQ score of 69 and the Vermont State Hospital superintendent's recommendation for her retention. She had wandered in and out of Vermont and had found herself in and out of public institutions. Between episodes of treatment in mental hospitals in Vermont and New York, she became pregnant, gave birth while in custody, married two years later, and subsequently abandoned her husband and child. She had worked as a model in another state and was believed by Abbott's sources to be sexually promiscuous. "At present Maggie is in a New York hospital undergoing treatment," Abbott reported, and will "probably be committed to some institution." Meanwhile her daughter had been rescued from the "disreputable people" with whom she had been left and, like her mother, had become a ward of the state of Vermont.[35]

Abbott had acquired the details of Maggie Simpson's personal life directly from the hospitals and welfare agencies that had provided services to Maggie. Abbott had requested the dates of confinement or services rendered, the reasons, and the precise cost to the institution or agency. Abbott's position as field-worker for the Eugenics Survey of Vermont was apparently sufficient to put her in the category of "need to know," for the replies were frank and prompt. Maggie Simpson, Abbott learned, had been hospitalized in New York for "hysteria." Medical examination revealed, however, that her apparent hysteria was brought on by abdominal pain in her right ovary or perhaps her appendix. After her appendectomy the hysterical symptoms had gone away.[36]

It is tempting to speculate that social workers and medical authorities had projected their own anxieties onto Maggie's diagnosis. If her appendectomy had been accompanied by sterilization, it would have allayed any concern on their part that she might become pregnant again. Maggie's history of institutionalization could account for her distress and apparent instability; she was one among a number of young women whom Abbott investigated most thoroughly and concluded that the system had neglected to protect.

Perkins concluded the second annual report with a table of the final cost estimates of the ten families selected for special study by the survey. The total, $225,650.05, amounted to less than the total amount the Eugenics Survey and the VCCL would ultimately spend surveying Vermont's human resources. The incidence of feeblemindedness and insanity in these families was noticeably low (5.6%), a fact Perkins attributed to counting only those whose condition had been verified by mental testing or whose symptoms were too extreme to require it. He noted that the survey had found many other "incompetents who 'are unable to handle their affairs with ordinary prudence' and are undoubtedly feebleminded," thus reinforcing the case for mental hygiene and eugenics remedies.

The "Eugenic Core" of the Vermont Commission on Country Life

The Vermont Commission on Country Life was formally constituted in May 1928. Its executive committee, chaired by Governor John Weeks, would provide the leadership and administration for seventeen committees comprising some two hundred volunteers and professionals dedicated to the improvement of rural conditions. Perkins, as secretary of the commission, would remain at the hub of its public and professional network within and outside the state and would manage, maintain, and finally inherit the records generated by the organization. Dr. Henry C. Taylor, a national figure in the field of rural sociology and economics, accepted the appointment of executive director that summer. The Social Science Research Council provided funds to organize the comprehensive rural survey. With their assistance the commission secured a substantial grant from the Laura Spelman Rockefeller Memorial Fund to finance the desired projects. Over the following year, Taylor and Perkins collaborated with the commission's executive committee to enlist many well-known local intellectuals and civic leaders to serve on various committees dedicated to preserving Vermont's natural beauty and to cultivating its agricultural and human resources. The Eugenics Survey would become the Committee on the Human Factor, with a special Subcommittee on the Care of Handicapped People.[37]

During his sabbatical, Perkins had made periodic trips to New York City to solicit advice and support from every possible funding agency as he developed his plans for the comprehensive rural survey. He was encouraged by the Social Science Research Council and the American Country Life Association to relinquish his emphasis on biological factors and stress sociological influences. His consultants at the Eugenics Record Office, however, urged him to assume a more active role in promoting mainline eugenics in the state. Arthur Estabrook, the Eugenic Record Office's most prominent rural eugenicist, advised Perkins to try to take over any family research of the Department of Public Welfare, co-opt the testing of schoolchildren begun by the National Committee on Mental Hygiene, and involve his organization in the courts by providing casework and psychological testing of defendants in felony and major misdemeanor trials. Whether or not Perkins realized it, he was caught in the midst of an escalating dialectic between sociologists and biologists over the authority and scientific merits of their study of the human condition. Both sides would produce more rigorous displays of hard scientific data (quantitative) not found in pedigrees or case histories that had characterized both eugenics and social work thus far. Like the American eugenicists, country life advocates were committed to the preservation and cultivation of the old pioneer stocks who they believed provided the leadership and conveyed the values of American institutions. Yet their solutions lay in the improvement of rural conditions, such as health care, education, and social life, to attract and retain young, well-educated Americans in agrarian communities. Eugenicists, having subordinated sociology to heredity and having gained visibility and power over public policy, were increasingly challenged by critics to provide more scientific evidence for their claims that attributed social problems to heredity.[38]

The nature-nurture issue arose in the deliberations of the newly formed executive committee of the Vermont Rural Survey as well. At its first meeting on May 18, 1928, Commissioner of Education Clarence Dempsey voiced skepticism over Perkins's assertion that rural Vermont stocks had declined in innate quality. Dempsey argued that the impact of rural poverty on the inadequate medical, social, and educational infrastructure of towns had produced the apparent degeneracy that Perkins attributed to heredity. In one remote country town having only twenty children, Dempsey had discovered that one boy had read every book in the library. The boy and his classmates were anxious for the library to add more books to its meager holdings. Beginning with the keynote speaker, Henry Israel of the American Country Life Association, every commentator at this first meeting of the VCCL executive committee advocated the need for improved rural services and cultural opportunities. While members of the executive committee expressed hearty gratitude for Perkins's efforts to organize and secure funds for the rural survey, his eugenic studies and his hereditarian assumptions seemed largely irrelevant to this group.[39]

All Perkins had to offer the VCCL was a failed attempt at a sterilization law, questionable progress on a census of feebleminded Vermonters living outside institutions, and a large volume of dubious genealogical data on defects in particular families and the public expense associated with their treatment. Perkins faced the disturbing possibility that his eugenics program and its underlying hereditarian assumptions might become marginalized in the commission he had created. To Perkins, who had never relinquished the naturalist orientation of his earlier training, the nature-nurture debate simply represented two sides of the same coin, and the family was the vector of both. As he explained in an address to Episcopal clergy in Burlington that September, "Being a biologist, I have been trained all my life to look for the interaction of factors in bringing about a stated result. Seldom in the animal world is it possible to study one special phase of the life of an organism profitably without taking into consideration the other phases as well. It has seemed to me the same thing applies with as much force to the study of the human animal."[40]

Perkins faced the dual challenge of reconciling the inherent antagonism between sociology and eugenics and providing scientific evidence to support that resolution. Perkins resorted to a familiar strategy not uncommon in the sciences and one for which he had a particular talent. He simply devised a new research plan to raise and presumably answer the question. He would then delegate its prosecution to his field staff, publicize whatever findings would enhance the political position of the survey, and claim discovery of new insights to replace previous positions he had taken.

Perkins was provided with an opportunity to shift his ground when he sought a new social worker to replace Conklin, who would be leaving in September to pursue a doctorate at the University of Pennsylvania. Perkins reported to his advisory committee that the organizations he had consulted wanted "something more scientific than our current data" and admitted, "It seems we have gone about as far as we are justified in going with general pedigree study that has occupied our attention hitherto."[41] He sought the advice of the Eugenics Survey advisory committee as well as of Charles Davenport about securing a new social worker with expertise in mental testing. In the end he hired a woman with no direct connection to the professional eugenics community. Mrs. Martha M. Wadman, a graduate of Mount Holyoke who had just completed a term as recorder and psychologist at Foxborough State Hospital, had the necessary experience in IQ testing to provide the quantitative evidence that the survey's earlier work lacked. In 1929, certainly, IQ tests qualified as hard, scientific data.

In order to salvage what he could from the genealogical studies and apply them to the questions that now appealed to the VCCL, Perkins drafted a new research plan for his advisory committee's approval and requested their "candid and merciless" criticisms concerning its value to the Committee on the Human Factor. The Eugenics Survey, he proposed, would conduct a reconnaissance of towns, classifying each according to its evident progress or decline. It would document demographic and economic trends and select representative towns in the state for more detailed study. To embed eugenics within the public history of the state, he devised the Key Family Study, in which the survey would correlate the social and economic history of selected towns with the quality and quantity of descendants of the town's founding families as revealed in genealogies. Towns suggested for study were relatively small (less than one thousand), composed primarily of the pioneer stocks of the state, and contained reliable informants willing to provide the necessary data to field-workers. That the towns "in decline" selected for study were ones inhabited by some of the "degenerate" families in the Eugenics Survey files comes as no surprise. They also lay in close proximity to the Green Mountain National Forest and near many tourist entry points to the state, where a display of "pockets of degeneracy" was out of character with the wholesome image of rural Vermont the state tourist board had been advertising. Martha Wadman began the study of key families in the small, declining towns of Readsboro and Sandgate in the southern part of the state, then proceeded to Lincoln in the Green Mountains. Perkins's new research plan, which he termed "eugenical-sociological," appealed to his advisors and his patron, Shirley Farr, who promised to fund the survey for the next three years with $6,000 per year.[42] Perkins's new approach not only marked a shift in the methods and interpretation of eugenics within Vermont, but it set the stage for a critical shift in Perkins's allegiances within the American eugenics movement as well.

The French Canadian Question

One area of eugenics research that Perkins had neglected but had not forgotten was the issue of race. Still inspired by Charles Davenport's suggestion that Vermont's "subnormalcy" arose from the replacement of native stock with French Canadians or other alien elements, Perkins hoped to make a sociological-eugenical study of "French Canadian Citizenship" as an integral part of the Comprehensive Rural Survey. In April 1928 he attempted to interest Charles Davenport in the idea. He asked Davenport to request the Genetics Division of the Carnegie Institution, which had funded rural eugenics projects, to detail Arthur Estabrook himself to Vermont for one year, at their expense, to do the study. Perkins may have sought Estabrook after reading a review of *The Win Tribe* published in the most recent issue of the *Journal of Heredity*; perhaps he sensed Estabrook might do something meaningful with the multiracial families, like the Gypsies, in the survey files.[43] Perkins informed Davenport that he had already written to Dr. Clark Wissler, an anthropologist at Columbia University, for help in developing a series of anthropometric tests to assess the degree of French Canadian extraction in sample populations in the northern and western regions of the state where French Canadians were especially numerous. The degree of French Canadian ancestry (full breed, half-breed, or quarter-breed) would then be correlated with data from mental testing, educational attainment, and various cultural factors, including the influence of Catholicism and the degree of participation in the social and civic life of the community. Perkins hinted that the National Committee on Mental Hygiene study would provide some very promising source material on French Canadian mental incompetence, which Estabrook would find most valuable. Davenport refused, suggesting that the Carnegie Institution could hardly be expected to supply the nation's leading expert in rural eugenics for a project of merely parochial relevance despite its possible academic merits. Moreover, at Carnegie's request, the Eugenics Record Office was abandoning survey work for "experimental" work in human heredity.[44]

Perkins continued to pressure Davenport to collaborate in the French Canadian study throughout the remainder of the year. Davenport politely and consistently declined to extend Carnegie Institution resources to the Vermont Commission on Country Life while encouraging Perkins to believe that the French Canadian question was worthy of eugenic study. In collaboration with Country Life Commission executive director Henry C. Taylor,

Perkins kept the issue of French Canadian replacement of native stocks on the agenda of the Committee on the Human Factor, hoping to incorporate it into geographical and population studies or insert it into the Committee on Religious Forces. But no plan concerning French Canadian Vermonters provided the eugenic focus that had attracted Perkins to the idea in the first place. In December 1928, Perkins made a final and futile attempt to enlist Davenport's cooperation to find a suitable field-worker to conduct the study. Davenport replied that the project would be an interesting one for a "vigorous young man" with an interest in eugenics. Davenport's question, "How much are you willing to pay a good man?" amounted to a refusal of any tangible support. It was also an implicit attack on Perkins's Eugenics Survey, which had been conducted solely by women.[45] Perkins never shared Davenport's attitudes toward women professionals. Yet Davenport's evident disdain for women eugenics workers, followed by his reassertion of Vermonters' alleged inferiority, rendered his refusal of help especially painful. Earlier that year, Perkins's star student, Laura Bliss, whose work on the physiology of twinning was precisely the sort of experimental work Davenport had encouraged, was refused a research position at the Eugenics Records Office, despite Perkins's effort on her behalf.[46]

Perkins informed Davenport that he hoped to find the right person to conduct the study at a negotiable salary, hinting that such an opportunity would be intrinsically attractive to a eugenicist:

> . . . It may not be wise to limit the ethnic studies to the French Canadian population alone. It is possible that racial derivations of sample areas in various parts of Vermont should be studied in order to get the best possible picture of the human factors in rural civilization. As you know, my reason for being particularly interested in the French Canadians is that they are so characteristically and so important a part of the population. They have been studied less than have European nationals. The problem is not unlike that of the Amerind invasion along the Mexican border.[47]

Davenport refused the bait. His reply was a slight, if not a downright insult. He knew of no qualified man for such an important project, as they were all actively employed in "important and remunerative" positions. He regretted the possibility that Perkins might not be able to proceed and added that the only reasons he could imagine for the "high defect rate in Vermont" was the replacement of emigrant native Vermonters with "some special alien stock," such as French Canadians or perhaps the Italian marble workers.[48]

In contrast to the Social Science Research Council, the American Country Life Association and their affiliates, the Carnegie-funded Eugenics Record Office had not shown the least interest in Perkins's broader vision of eugenics, with its synthesis of mental hygiene and rural sociology. But when Davenport raised once more the specter of Vermont's embarrassment at the draft boards, the assault on Perkins's pride would be Davenport's last. Perkins dispensed with Davenport as a mentor. To do so, he used the results of the NCMH study of schoolchildren, which challenged every suggestion Davenport had made but had refused to provide the means to pursue. Perkins's response to Davenport addressed only the issue of Vermont subnormalcy. The NCMH study, he wrote, "showed no larger proportion of subnormal children in rural and urban schools than have been reported from various other states." Not only that, but the study showed, for racial differences, "that the incidence of subnormalcy was almost exactly the same among families of foreign origin as amongst those of native stock."[49]

Perkins's admission of this new evidence suggests that he had neglected to study the data closely in his enthusiasm to identify French Canadian inferiority or had previously ignored data that did not fit his assumptions. More likely he had suppressed the findings concerning families of foreign origin in the hope of Carnegie support. He provided it now only to challenge Davenport to defend his allegations about Vermont's low ranking at the draft boards.[50] In reply, Davenport suggested that the Vermont draft boards had been to blame for the discrepancy (not his analysis) in perhaps making excessively rigid selections and eliminating those with the slightest defect. Perkins never replied to Davenport's final insult and suspended correspondence with the Eugenics Record Office for the next three years. He would not correspond with Davenport again regarding the Eugenics Survey until 1936, when Perkins's assistant director, Elin Anderson, would expose the prejudice in Davenport's assertions.[51]

Perkins never again mentioned his original plan to study French Canadian Vermonters. His decision to abandon the explicitly eugenic French Canadian study was opportune. Opposition to this sort of race research among respected biologists was mounting. That year Davenport's own scientific reputation would be sacrificed over his treatment of race in his controversial and much criticized study, *Race Crossing in Jamaica*.[52] But Perkins did not take a decisive stand on the other side either. Had he truly embraced the scientific integrity he claimed for the Eugenics Survey and publicized the data he had confided to Davenport, he might have changed the course of Vermont history and his place within it. Instead, he remained conspicuously silent on the NCMH findings, missing the opportunity to openly challenge the widespread prejudice in Vermont against French Canadians and other ethnic groups. While the findings of the NCMH were used by the VCCL Committee on the Handicapped, the Department of Education, and the Brandon State School for the Feebleminded, Perkins chose to ignore them for the next decade.[53]

A More Positive Approach: Vermont's "Fitter Families"

In January, Perkins also had to confront the sterilization issue, as the biennial legislative session was about to begin. The success of the VCCL required public trust in the Eugenics Survey as an apolitical, nonsectarian, and purely scientific enterprise, and its previous promotion of sterilization had compromised that identity. Perkins requested the Eugenics Survey advisory committee's "permission to refrain for the present from carrying out your instructions" of promoting sterilization during the 1929 biennial legislative session. Referring to the 1927 failed attempt to pass a sterilization law and the likelihood that the issue would surface again, Perkins feared that his explicit support would jeopardize the entire VCCL: "It is important that nothing arouse suspicion among any important group, economic, social, political, or religious. In order to secure as complete cooperation as possible it may be better for the Eugenics Survey to avoid antagonizing some people who have strong convictions on the sterilization question. This need not hamper any of you, but perhaps I had better keep out of it."[54] Perkins's timing was significant. He sent this request the day before his final overture to Davenport regarding his hopes for the French Canadian study, leaving little doubt about which "social, religious, political, and economic group" he was most worried about offending. His advisors agreed and apparently avoided the issue themselves, for no bill was introduced in the legislature that year. Instead, Perkins prepared another annual report to emphasize the new direction the Eugenics Survey had taken.[55]

In his third annual report, issued in February 1929, Perkins attempted to re-create the Eugenics Survey as an integral component of the Vermont Commission on Country Life and secure its role as a sympathetic authority over local social matters. At the same time, he used it as an opportunity to rid himself of the albatross of "negative eugenics," which had been criticized by some members of his advisory committee after his assault on the Doolittle clan.[56] To this end, Perkins placed his first two reports in historical perspective, acknowledging that the *original* purpose for surveying "low grade families" had been, first, to gather and classify "facts having a clear bearing upon social betterment problems in Vermont . . . for future reference by legitimate organizations, state departments, and authorized social workers." Second, the survey had sought source material for the scientific study of the role of heredity that bore directly on the social welfare of Vermont. Perkins reiterated the survey's purely scientific and impartial motivation, as evidenced by its association with the university and the favorable reception its research had received "among scientific workers in the field of human heredity all over the country."[57] To absolve himself of responsibility for the bill for eugenic sterilization, Perkins relegated it to the past:

. . . *Early in the history* of the Survey, the Advisory Committee went on record
as favoring the passage of certain laws looking toward the improvement of the
population of Vermont by some restrictive measure. The Survey was first conceived as a means of applying scientific technique to the question of the wisdom of such measures. The results have in no way lessened the faith of the
Committee in such laws, but the scope of the Survey has greatly broadened so
that any particular form of legislation no longer constitutes its chief purpose. It
became apparent *early in the history of the enterprise* that its scope was much
broader than that.[58] (emphasis mine)

Explaining away the previous reports as "history" enabled Perkins to create a new public image of the Eugenics Survey—as the Committee on the
Human Factor of the Vermont Commission on Country Life. Concealing his
own role as instigator of the campaign for sterilization by attributing it to his
advisory committee was a bold move and shows how clearly he understood
the tenuousness of his position. Except for his report on additional cross-
indexing, clock-dial charts, and the development of a file called "English Cor-
ruptions of French Names," each major section of the third annual report
contributed to this renegotiation of the purpose of eugenics in Vermont.

First, Perkins reprinted "The Children of Feebleminded and Insane Parents," an analysis of one of Francis Conklin's statistical compilations of the
pedigree data, which had been published the previous year in *Eugenical
News*. The report served several purposes. For one thing, the mathematical
approach submerged the deeply personal nature of their investigations
within an apparently more scientific format. Second, Conklin's statistics enabled Perkins to situate the survey's findings within the most recent eugenics
research, particularly Paul Popenoe's studies showing that the fecundity of
the feebleminded had been exaggerated in the past. Third, Conklin's compu-
tations helped to put the draft board results to rest, while promoting the desirability of reproductive interventions. (See fig. 3.2.) Conklin had found that
Vermont's feebleminded and insane persons reproduced at the same or a
lower rate than elsewhere in the nation (3.5 children per "inadequate" family) but still at a higher rate than parents "not known to be feebleminded or
insane" (who averaged 3.04 children per family). The graph quantified *visu-
ally* information that Perkins knew, by his own admission, to be unreliable
and unscientific. The data had been collected from Harriett Abbott's "face
sheets" that determined insanity or feeblemindedness from institutional records and informants' opinions, not from psychiatric testing. Perkins may have
accomplished a more important goal in this essay. The mathematical approach delivered the old eugenic message in a revised, impersonal form:
insane or feebleminded parents posed a great risk to unborn children, especially if they mated with others having the same tendencies. The problem of

mental defect in Vermont, previously embodied in the Pirates and Gypsies, town idiots, and families known to all in every town, was now reduced to a set of statistical abstractions on a graph.[59]

In a second article, "The Study of Better Branches: The Rector Family," Perkins attempted to dissociate the survey from its previous negative rhetoric and present a more nuanced view of Vermont families and their contributions to their communities (fig. 3.3). He nevertheless preserved the eugenic duality of "social" individuals—"those who are apparently law abiding, self-supporting and doing some useful work"—and "unsocial" persons, who displayed the familiar repertoire of pathologies.[60] The great discovery in the Rector family, previously categorized as one of the original degenerate ones, was that all the asocial types were descendants of one insane son, Asa, and his allegedly insane wife. (Asa and his wife were of old colonial stock; Asa's parents had moved to Vermont from Connecticut in the eighteenth century.) Of Asa's eight siblings, the descendants of six were unknown and therefore not open to hypothetical assessment. Two of Asa's siblings, however, had generated diverse, intelligent, and highly competent families with no indication of any defect. For the most part, the Rectors had contributed constructively to Vermont communities in various capacities—as business owners, as professionals, and as farmers, foresters, and skilled and day laborers. Even Asa's

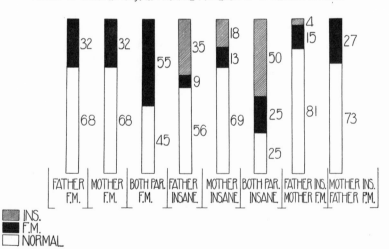

3.2 Francis Conklin's statistical summary of Vermont's "eugenical problem."
"The Children of Feebleminded and Insane Parents," *Third Annual Report of the Eugenics Survey of Vermont*, 1929. Courtesy Special Collections Department, University of Vermont Library.

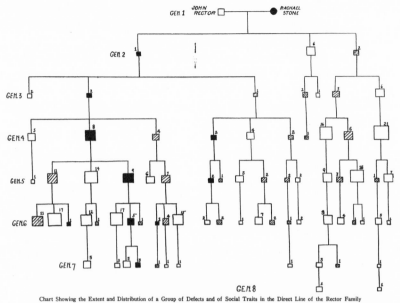

Chart Showing the Extent and Distribution of a Group of Defects and of Social Traits in the Direct Line of the Rector Family

The symbols here used—black for unsocial, cross hatching for social, and white for undetermined individuals—are the same as in the condensed chart, and the use of the terms is as explained at the beginning of the article on the Rector family. For purposes of compactness, the individuals are grouped as far as possible, the size of the square agreeing with the number against it and indicating the number of persons included.

3.3 The "Rectors," initially one of the Eugenics Survey's "degenerate" families, were transformed in a survey of their "better branches" into a "normal," socially diverse Vermont family. This revision enabled Perkins to adjust his "fact-finding" reports in response to criticism of the earlier style of family research. *Third Annual Report of the Eugenics Survey of Vermont*, 1929. Courtesy Special Collections Department, University of Vermont Library.

deviant and unemployed descendants had produced more accomplished, intelligent Rectors, with excellent character, than deficient ones, thereby compensating the community for the "heavy cost to support delinquent and deficient individuals from the same stock."[61]

Perkins took this opportunity to teach a revised eugenics lesson. Family worth, both from a eugenic point of view and from his survey's own research, would not be measured in terms of wealth or social standing but in terms of the diversity of talent, interests, and contributions to community life. Every family, the survey had found, had unfortunate members, and even the most asocial families produced valuable, notable children. Normal families displayed a broad range of traits; therefore, the presence of mental incompetence in a family should not detract from the reputation of the family as a whole. In Perkins's refinement of his previous strategy of condemning entire families as a "social and moral drag" on the community, he artfully finessed any criticism his earlier reports might have engendered. The sterilization controversies were not far from his mind, however, as he concluded the Rector case study: "This is not to be taken as offsetting any arguments advocating measures for the restriction of propagation of defectives. It is probable that no competent board of examiners would have recommended these people in the better branches for sterilization."[62]

In a third piece, Martha Wadman's study of the Furman family showcased the sort of work the Eugenics Survey would be doing in its new capacity as the Committee on the Human Factor of the VCCL. Perkins introduced his "eugenical-sociological" approach with the question "What part has heredity been playing in the rise and growth and, in many cases cause the decline of rural communities in Vermont?" "Our basic thesis is this: The families that live in a town for several generations make their mark, for both good and ill, upon the town. They help or hinder its own growth and give it their own moral, intellectual and social tone. Most families, perhaps all, both add and detract from the welfare of their communities. Their contributions may be measured as regards the past, and predicted for the future in terms of their more positive *hereditary* traits, whether these are predominantly constructive or social, or destructive—antisocial."[63]

The Furmans had been among the earliest settlers in the Quaker town of "Garfield" (Lincoln) which was established in 1798. Matthew Furman, the first town blacksmith and later the town's miller, had contributed to the growth of Garfield in both wealth and descendants. Many of the 372 persons in the Furman "tribe" were scattered across the country, yet they still retained their family connections and pride in their ancestry. The Furman narrative, embellished with touching anecdotes of Quaker "industry, thrift, and simple living," focused on the Furmans' continued distinction and achievements in other parts of the country. The story played on a well-known image of Vermont as the ancestral home, while presenting a new profile of the healthy, wholesome, normal Vermont family—socially diverse with occasional "defects" (insanity and suicidal tendencies in the case of the Furmans). (See fig. 3.4.) Garfield ranked among the endangered communities in Vermont, however, a fact Perkins linked to the emigration and lack of replacement of Furmans or others like them in town.[64]

The Furman piece was a prelude to the extensive studies of Vermont towns, families, and migration patterns that would appear in the fourth and fifth annual reports. In the fourth annual report (March 1930), Perkins profiled another "normal, healthy, Vermont family," the Burrs of Garfield. The Burrs had a typical share of handicaps (epilepsy, deafness, mental deficiency, and insanity) yet were generally well adjusted and had made important contributions throughout the history of the state in the usual diverse occupations

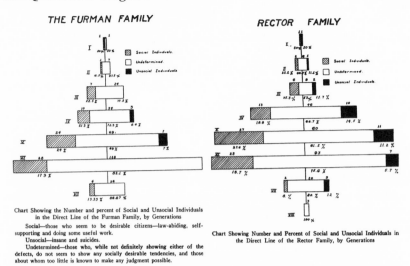

THE FURMAN FAMILY

RECTOR FAMILY

Chart Showing the Number and percent of Social and Unsocial Individuals
in the Direct Line of the Furman Family, by Generations

Social—those who seem to be desirable citizens—law-abiding, self-
supporting and doing some useful work.
Unsocial—insane and suicides.
Undetermined—those who, while not definitely showing either of the
defects, do not seem to show any socially desirable tendencies, and those
about whom too little is known to make any judgment possible.

Chart Showing Number and Percent of Social and Unsocial Individuals in
the Direct Line of the Rector Family, by Generations

3.4 Despite the emphasis on the positive contributions of these families, the eugenic
goal of sorting people according to their desirability and assumed value to society
characterized all eugenics research and publication. *Third Annual Report of the Eugenics
Survey of Vermont*, 1929. Courtesy Special Collections Department, University of Vermont Library.

and their distinguished record of public service. No reference was made to
hereditary degeneracy; the handicaps found were not a general pattern but
were isolated events concentrated in "one small branch" in a few generations.
The survey was pleased to report that these descendants of Vermont's early
settlers were holding their own yet lamented their loss of influence due to
outmigration and declining birthrates. The challenges the Burrs faced in
farming the rocky soil in their mountain town testified to their rugged spirit
and illustrated a key factor driving the rural exodus. The Burrs who left, in
Wadman's and Perkins's judgment, had made the eugenic choice. They
demonstrated their adaptability and initiative, and as a result, the Burrs "have
not crowded themselves into Garfield where they would have intermarried
and become enervated for want of work." Moreover, one town's loss was another's gain. Those who remained behind had also made a commendable
choice, one of commitment to family, farm, and community.[65]

Perkins's synthesis of eugenics (genealogy) and social history would enable
a broad-minded eugenicist to see the eugenic core of their research and a sociologist to see a plan for improved opportunities grounded in social science
theory and practice. His celebration of Vermont traditions and the heterogeneity of Vermont families was politically astute, for he avoided offending

his broadening constituency in Vermont while maintaining the eugenic core of the VCCL's survey of Vermont population trends. But Perkins's town and key family studies added a local historical dimension to his eugenics vision, which he made explicit in the mission statement of the Committee on the Human Factor: to connect the environmental, economic, and social factors in rural Vermont to the liabilities and assets of its people and "to use the experience of the state and the heritage of her rural citizens as a guide in building a program for the state." For patriotic Vermonters to whom Perkins made his appeal, the preservation of the state's beloved past had been turned into an exercise in eugenics.[66]

Perkins's family profiles in the third and fourth annual reports emerged at a time when the American Eugenics Society, through the efforts of its zealous executive secretary, Leon Whitney, was sponsoring "Fitter Family" contests at state fairs and contests for the best sermon on eugenics by inspired preachers. The official publication of the American Eugenics Society, *Eugenics*, also catered to a popular audience with politically and religiously charged articles on population control and family life. While Whitney's populist approach played well to audiences at state fairs in the Midwest, it ran counter to internal changes within the American eugenics establishment, where efforts were underway to refashion eugenics research and education into a more scientific, intellectually driven enterprise. Eugenicists at Harvard, Yale, and Johns Hopkins, for example, were shifting the focus of eugenics research from the idea of "better breeding" to more rigorous research on population trends— quantitative assessments of the effects of social and economic trends on mate selection and birthrates, and studies of the interaction of heredity and environmental influences. Whitney's promotional schemes were becoming a liability to the scientific image these scientists wanted to project.[67]

Perkins's new family studies, in contrast, provided a more nuanced view of the "eugenic family" set in the context of its history and its ongoing relationship to the community. His connection of these factors with family size and community opportunities for Vermont's youth also set the family profiles more securely within the goals of the country life movement. His family histories were more in character with the attempt to investigate hereditary factors and reproductive trends within their social environment—that is, to think of human populations as natural ones to be studied and cultivated as such, rather than an experiment in domestic breeding. While Perkins's family profiles, from our perspective, were heavily biased, political, and lacking in scientific rigor, neither he nor his contemporaries placed them in the same category as Leon Whitney's "Fitter Family" contests. Perkins's new eugenic family narratives reflected a newfound conservatism, common sense, and a greater sensitivity to the complex and ambiguous factors that influenced human life.[68]

Institutional Investigations:
The "3 D's" as Handicapped and at Risk

While the problems of dependency, delinquency, and mental deficiency were rapidly receding from the public portrait of Vermont family life, they were not forgotten. They had become the particular mission of a special subcommittee of the VCCL's Committee on the Human Factor, the Subcommittee on the Care of the Handicapped, whose mission was to survey needs of Vermont's social problem group and evaluate the quality of services provided for their care. Chaired by the general secretary of the Vermont Children's Aid Society, L. Josephine Webster, the subcommittee consisted of the Eugenics Survey advisory committee members representing state institutions in the Department of Public Welfare and the state correctional facilities—the same leaders in progressive reform who had been urging the state to adopt a comprehensive program of mental testing, reporting, and managing Vermont's mentally handicapped population. Martha Wadman, in her official role of Eugenics Survey investigator, applied her expertise in psychometrics to study the needs of target populations in institutional settings for the Subcommittee on the Care of the Handicapped. In 1929 she studied the women inmates at the Riverside Reformatory in Rutland and conducted follow-up case work on the Brandon waiting list (persons referred to the State School for the Feebleminded who had been denied admittance because of limited available space). Perkins published her results in the fourth annual report (1930). Both studies reflected the new, more clinical approach to eugenics—an approach that replaced family histories and pedigree analysis with individual case work and statistical studies of "handicapped" individuals and groups.

Lena Ross, Eugenics Survey advisory committee member and superintendent of the Reformatory for Women in Rutland, had suggested a study of her inmates to determine the extent to which they owed their circumstances to mental subnormalcy. Superintendent Ross had been providing special accommodations and follow-up supervision for drug-addicted inmates and believed "feebleminded female sex offenders" deserved a similar program of rehabilitation. Perkins and Ross felt the project was of eugenic significance, for it would afford more protection to society, to the women themselves, and to their children, who would "presumably share in the antisocial proclivities of their mothers."[69]

Using the Stanford Revision of the Binet-Simon Scale, Wadman tested the fifty-three women inmates, including sixteen recidivists, and compiled statistics on the nature of their offenses, their ages, educational attainment in school, form of employment, marital status, and number of children. Wadman claimed to have ignored the family history and social background of these women (which previous eugenics work had emphasized). Yet her report actually lent more rigorous support to the theory that mental deficiency (carefully measured and presumably innate) was responsible to a large degree for the circumstances of these women. Wadman recast the stereotype of the "feebleminded" woman in a less personal, yet more compelling, display of statistical data. Wadman admitted her sample of women recidivists was too small to make a "fair comparison" of their IQ levels with those of first offenders. Yet she reported statistical patterns that confirmed Superintendent Ross's initial assumptions about such women. Women recidivists showed a lower distribution of IQ in comparison with the general population, with an average mental age of ten to eleven years. Compared to the first offenders, the recidivists had dropped out of school sooner and were more frequently arrested for sexual delinquency and petty theft. They had been predominantly employed as unskilled labor in domestic, hotel, and restaurant services, rather than in factories, stores, or more carefully supervised work environments.[70]

Wadman used her findings to argue on behalf of the vulnerability of these women. Her statistics created a new profile of the incompetent mother, who required protection, advocacy, special training, and close supervision. Most of the recidivists, Wadman found, had been incarcerated for "crimes of submission or crimes of imperfect emotional control" (ten of the sixteen recidivists were serving time for sex offenses or breach of parole for previous sex offenses, mostly adultery, but also lewd and lascivious conduct, prostitution, or having sex when infected with venereal disease).[71] The term of confinement was too short to successfully retrain "mentally-deficient sex-delinquent" women, who "are released only to return in a short time, either pregnant or having borne illegitimate children during their short period of freedom." The problem, Wadman concluded, was the failure of the judicial system, which condemned such women as immoral and punished them for their mental handicap. Their convictions for petty larceny, adultery, and breach of parole were rooted in ignorance and lack of foresight, not malice. The women, Wadman argued, should be treated as hospital patients, not criminals, and given special vocational training, community supervision, and protection from their own vulnerabilities to the charms of unprincipled men. Citing the generally low IQ of the incarcerated women and their rather minor offenses, Wadman surmised that they were not typical of the general female delinquent population. She thus reinforced the incompetency argument by suggesting that "only the less clever ones 'get caught.'"[72]

The child welfare theme was also restated statistically, showing that the women in the Riverside Reformatory had, on the average, 3.9 children. Because of their mothers' incarceration, 154 children were living in broken homes, foster care, or state institutions. Wadman worried about what would become of them: "since we must guard the future as well as care for the present, our deepest concern is to help these children who are deprived of the most important social influence in life, a good home. It is left so much to chance what will become of them."[73]

Perkins's eclectic eugenics program for Vermont had, since its inception, promoted a comprehensive state program of mental testing, registration of mental defectives, and the expansion of special classes and vocational training for the feebleminded. The Rutland Reformatory study restated the need for all of these reforms and, most important, to show the Eugenics Survey and its associated agencies as *advocates* of such women, whose needs were clinical and best understood by qualified psychiatrists and psychiatric social workers rather than by well-meaning yet uninformed lay persons. Sterilization of such women was never mentioned in the Riverside Reformatory study, but all the essential innuendos were supplied.[74]

Martha Wadman's case studies of persons on the Brandon waiting list exemplified the growing interest of psychiatric social workers in hearing their clients' own stories and providing support for their adjustment within the community. This project had been inspired by Wadman's discovery of a woman who had been referred to Brandon a number of years previously, was refused admittance, and had become an apparently well-adjusted wife and mother in the interim. She wrote to Dr. Truman Allen, superintendent of the Brandon Training School, to ask his opinion on the further study of such cases. Perhaps the waiting list would reveal that referrals to Brandon had been too hastily made or that feeblemindedness had been too casually diagnosed. Perhaps many feebleminded persons could adjust satisfactorily to society, despite their handicaps, without the special training at Brandon.[75]

Despite Wadman's hopeful attitude and concern for the well-being of the Brandon referrals, the manner in which Perkins published three of her cases showed little optimism or sympathy. The parents or guardians of the young people in question were not blamed for the problems found but were depicted as doing their best with inadequate state support or special services in their communities. Perkins's sensational titles may have provoked the old eugenic anxieties. "Tom, a Town Charge," "Allen, an Idiot, Mars a Normal Home," and "Mary, a Potential Sex-Delinquent" portrayed the need for early diagnosis of mental and emotional instability, the uncertain prognosis for normal social adjustment, and the disruption of normal family and community life caused by insufficient professional intervention in the care of socially or mentally handicapped persons.[76]

Tom, a grade school dropout with a history of foster care, worked as a farm laborer for families with an apparent interest in his welfare. No longer a town charge, Tom was an attractive, tall, slim, and gregarious youth, resentful of his standing in the community, resistant of his employers' efforts to teach him responsibility, and unaccepting "of his own limitations." Seven-year-old

Allen, severely handicapped from polio, required intensive care that had made his mother a nervous wreck, had ruined her marriage, and had forced her to place her two younger children in the care of relatives. Mary, the "Potential Sex-delinquent," provided a portrait of the problem Wadman profiled in the women at the Riverside Reformatory. Mary had dropped out of school at age sixteen in the third grade. Local authorities had tried unsuccessfully to gain her parents' permission to send her to the Brandon state school, despite her IQ of 54.6 and her "trouble in school from the sex standpoint." Mary had been hired in domestic service by three "very patient, understanding women in the community" and subsequently fired for her "unpleasant behavior." Mary's "low mentality, an uncontrollable temper and abnormal interest in sex," according to this report, put her at serious risk of coming "to the attention of the State authorities, if not for mental deficiency, then for delinquency." Mental deficiency, whatever its cause or severity, these cases illustrated, could disrupt family and community life. The Brandon waiting list cases supported the desired initiatives to expand the facilities at Brandon and to provide traveling child guidance and psychiatric clinics, staffed with professional social workers who could supervise young persons likely to become dependent or delinquent themselves and unsuitable parents for the next generation of Vermonters.

In the fourth annual report, Perkins realigned his eugenics education with the latest consensus in genetics by pointing out one of the frequent "misconceptions" about eugenics: "Defects do not actually breed out ever. But they may be kept in abeyance indefinitely by favorable matings." Critics of eugenics had refuted the extravagant claims of mainline eugenicists by mathematical demonstrations that recessive genes (and their resulting conditions) could never be eliminated through restricting reproduction of those who evidently bore them. Many eugenicists, like Perkins, were backing off from their previous positions by casting the new "truth" as an expression of their own progressive, scientific outlook. Human race improvement, Perkins argued, would rest on enlightened mate selection. Special training for some of the mentally handicapped would improve their chances for a favorable match. He urged parents and family members to seek guidance from professional experts and rehabilitation services for handicapped children as one means to better their situation.[77]

Perkins concluded the fourth annual report with five pages of tables summarizing the data drawn from the records of the original fifty-five family pedigrees. The charts served as reminders of the enduring presence of feeblemindedness, Huntington's chorea and other forms of insanity, tuberculosis, alcoholism, and the other traits that had once characterized Vermont "degeneracy." Devoid of such personal designations as Pirate, Gypsy, or Doolittle, the fifty-five families in 1930 had become nothing more than numbers in a table, whose significance to the survey was conveyed in the past tense. The targets of reproductive intervention were no longer specific families known to the community but particular traits. The table reminded Vermonters of the unchecked presence of particular "defects" in Vermont that warranted attention but in strictly therapeutic, clinical settings under the supervision of qualified professionals. The depersonalization of the social problem group may have enabled some hesitant politicians to support legalized eugenic sterilization.[78]

By 1930 interest in Goddard's feeblemindedness theory, from the eugenic standpoint, had waned; its complex etiology was confirmed and becoming more rigorously studied. The term "mental deficiency" replaced "feeble-mindedness" even in Perkins's literature. The Brandon State School for the Feebleminded became the Brandon Training School in 1929, and the VCCL Subcommittee on the Handicapped hoped to enlist the support of parents in early diagnosis of disabilities in their children. By 1930, Perkins had carefully positioned the Eugenics Survey as an advocate for "normal" diversity of Vermont families, whose variability provided the raw material for rural renewal. He avoided the French Canadian question as well. While a desire to promote Vermont as a distinctly "American" state and Vermonters as the "fitter families" of old New England stocks might explain Perkins's silence on the matter of race, I am inclined to think that his reticence was a symptom of his confusion and his habitual caution during periods of uncertainty. Race research was becoming a liability and source of dissension among biologists. Perkins, a consensus follower, chose to watch the debate rather than participate in it. As population studies displaced family studies in eugenics research, Perkins gradually adjusted his research and publicity accordingly. Quantification of human problems and social trends provided a more impersonal and less controversial tool to explore eugenic questions.[79]

Perkins's departure from his earlier eugenics strategies impressed at least one noted American biologist, who, like Perkins, was retreating from his previous strong hereditarian assumptions. Harvard geneticist William E. Castle wrote to Perkins in high praise of the survey's progress: "Each Report seems to me increasingly valuable. I have read this one cover to cover, and wish to express my admiration of its clarity of statement, freedom from sweeping generalizations, its judicial and common sense attitude toward both negative and positive agencies. I wish you success in the further prosecution of this important work."[80]

Perkins's efforts were appreciated in Vermont as well. His colleagues had been sufficiently impressed with his efforts on behalf of families and children to include him in the Vermont delegation to President Hoover's White House Conference on Child Health and Protection, in which the "Child's Bill of Rights" was drafted.

Rural Renewal: Elin Anderson

In September 1929, Martha Wadman resigned and returned to Massachusetts to resume graduate studies. Now that the Eugenics Survey was functioning in a subordinate capacity within the VCCL Committee on the Human Factor, Perkins sought a field assistant with expertise in rural sociology and a commitment to the country life philosophy. Perkins interviewed six promising applicants in New York City and selected Elin Anderson. A native of Winnipeg with five years of high school teaching experience in Canadian schools, Anderson had just received a master's degree from the New York School of Social Work.[81] Anderson brought the survey unprecedented national distinction over the next seven years, as she applied her training and interest in sociology to the questions of the eugenic significance of the rural exodus and ethnic relations. Her investigations enabled Perkins to inscribe the VCCL with the core ideology of eugenics. Her sociological approach would turn these issues into a population problem whose solution lay in community organization and interaction.

At the New York School of Social Work, Anderson had become a disciple of the community organization movement through the influence of one of her professors, Eduard Lindeman. Lindeman had criticized the "scientific management" approach to social work, arguing that it had converted social workers into bureaucratic functionaries who simply dispensed prescriptions for social rehabilitation by assessing symptoms and processing clients through the channels of bureaucratic machinery. Social workers had paid little attention to the client's own story, feelings, or personal aspirations. Lindeman and his like-minded colleagues sought to decentralize, democratize, and humanize social agencies through the concept of cooperative democracy. Direct participation in civic affairs and the creation of neighborhood or community-based institutions by the collaboration of the residents themselves, they argued, would rejuvenate democracy and enable each citizen to realize his or her own potential. Individual self-realization and community solidarity were the defining themes of the community organization movement. The social worker in this context served as a mediator and facilitator of the overall mission. He or she would study and analyze the sources of divisiveness and the personal attitudes of community members while at the same time promoting involvement in community enterprises. The public school, the Grange, and other nonsectarian, community-sponsored programs would turn citizens into neighbors. Such organizations could free the people from manipulation by competing special interest groups—religious, social, or political—each claiming to represent the interests of particular identifiable segments of the community. Community solidarity would replace old allegiances. In Ameri-

can cities the community organization movement took the form of neighborhood associations, while rural American towns and villages—with the help of
grants from the Rockefeller Foundation, the Social Science Research Council, and similar organizations—surveyed needs and experimented with progressive community programs.[82]

For Anderson, part of the appeal of the cooperative democracy model
may have been rooted in her memory of the 1919 Winnipeg general strike
just prior to her senior year at the University of Manitoba. Its climax in the
massacre of Winnipeg citizens by the Royal Canadian Mounted Police may
have impressed her with the power of special interest groups to foment race
and class hostilities and transform community feeling into violence and
bloodshed. The VCCL presented her with an opportunity to conduct meaningful research in support of community building and to serve as an influential mediator. Perkins sensed that Anderson would provide precisely what
the Eugenics Survey needed to enhance its importance within the commission and to place its investigations within the traditions, vision, and history of
the state.[83]

Perkins assigned Anderson the project of relating migration to the eugenic
prognosis of three rural towns in Vermont, one "in decline" (Jamaica), one in
renewal and growth (Waitsfield), and a well-kept agrarian community (Cornwall), where French Canadian farmers were gradually replacing the old Vermont stock. Waitsfield, not far from the state capital, had been suggested for
study as "the best town in Washington County." It demonstrated economic
and social progress in contrast to neighboring towns nestled in the Green
Mountains. A number of notable Vermonters had been born there, and
twenty-five Waitsfield families could trace their ancestry back nine generations, to the original settlers in the eighteenth century. Jamaica was selected
as the town in decline because its residents had invested little effort in keeping up the town. "Wild and picturesque, beautiful and not developed as a
summer place," VCCL leaders viewed this town on the southeast edge of the
Green Mountain Forest as an ideal spot for tourist and recreational development, if only it could be made presentable.[84]

Anderson published her findings in the Eugenics Survey's fifth annual report, *Selective Migration from Three Rural Vermont Towns and Its Significance*, the longest, most developed of any of the Eugenics Survey's publications. She combined sociological analysis with local history in a way that
would define Vermont studies for decades to come. To assess the eugenic or
dysgenic prognosis for rural Vermont towns, Anderson studied the town histories, town clerks' records, grand lists, and vital statistics of Waitsfield, Cornwall, and Jamaica. She lived in each town for eight weeks, became acquainted
with every family, and interviewed residents and emigrants. She participated
in town activities and absorbed the general ambience and the particular char-

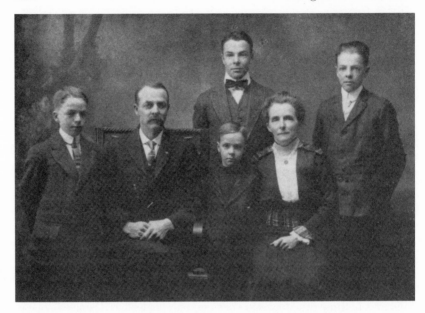

3.5 Elin Anderson sustained the eugenic link between family quality and community
progress in rural Vermont. "A Pomona family, whose sons have gone away. One has become a mechan-
ical engineer, one a full professor at Princeton University, and the other a university instructor. The youngest
remains to help carry on the home farm which has been in the family since 1865." Elin Anderson, *Selective
Migration from Three Rural Vermont Towns and its Significance. Fifth Annual Report of the Eugenics Survey
of Vermont,* 1931. Courtesy Special Collections Department, University of Vermont Library.

acter of each town and its people. Anderson's work, while based in rural sociology, still supported Perkins's desire to use the quality and quantity of the
"Old American" families in each town as an index of their eugenic value.
What emerged was a profile, not of specific families but of the eugenic or dysgenic community, classified according to its ability to attract, sustain, and cultivate fertile, healthy, enterprising, and well-educated families.[85]

All three towns, Anderson found, had been affected by the rural exodus,
showing a marked decline in one age group (15–45 years). All continued to be
dominated by Vermont Yankee families; immigrant replacement shared an
ethnic and social heritage similar to those who left, with only a 4 percent sub-
stitution of "foreign for native stock."[86] Those leaving for more urban areas
tended to be more educated. Anderson's interviews indicated that emigrants
had moved primarily for economic reasons. Those who remained had expressed a greater investment in family and community, remaining content
with their limited opportunities locally and the necessary reduction in their
standard of living. (See fig. 3.5.) While it may have been comforting to old

Vermonters that their ancestral stock continued to dominate rural Vermont, its vulnerability to future decline and redistribution to nonrural areas was worrisome. In response to such anxieties, Anderson's comparison of the three towns provided a basis for remedies of these dysgenic trends.

Anderson found "Pomona" (Waitsfield) to have the most potential. Not only was it situated in a protected valley surrounded by serene mountains, but it was well kept, moderately prosperous, and generously supportive of the local school despite rising taxes. Most important, in Anderson's view, its citizens were "keenly interested in the affairs of their town." The major threat to the preservation of the character of the town and the "excellent class of people" who lived there was the immigration of "inferior types." Anderson noted that this element consisted not of foreigners but of lower-class native Vermonters who had been hired as farm laborers or lumberjacks. They had found permanent accommodation in "the shabbiest homes," and, Anderson noticed, their standards of honesty and morality failed to measure up to the standards of the rest of the town. Anderson concluded that Waitsfield was basically eugenic and recommended a reduction in the tax burden to support schools and to expand recreational activities for its youth.[87]

"Beaufield" (Cornwall) was almost entirely agricultural. It had maintained its integrity and self-sufficiency despite the rural exodus of old Vermont stocks and their replacement by French-Canadian farming families. Though the population had declined and community solidarity was challenged by language and religious barriers, French Canadian and Yankee farmers cooperated in Grange activities, in civic affairs, and in keeping "out of their town persons of questionable character, or people who may become dependent on the town." Anderson may have used Beaufield to demonstrate her belief that ethnic diversity was eugenic when persons of different nationalities cooperated in the interest of community self-sufficiency and improvement. Yet her concern over (dysgenic) ethnic prejudice in Vermont surfaced when she pointed out that many "old residents" respected the French Canadian immigrants but regretted that their town was no longer "one big family" and predicted that many of their farms would eventually be abandoned or sold to French Canadians.[88]

Anderson's opinion surveys confirmed that migration was largely a matter of "self-selection." Those who had abandoned marginal lands did so as an expression of an innate restlessness, ambition, and greater desire for the social and economic opportunities in more vital towns and urban centers. In the declining rural town, "Sylvania" (Jamaica), Anderson found few incentives to attract or retain such people. Its citizens were less intellectual, less ambitious, and content to "just get by." Anderson's photographs and descriptions of Sylvania's village and farms reinforced the linkage between "the human factor" and rural decline. (See fig. 3.6.) Very little land was cultivated, more farms

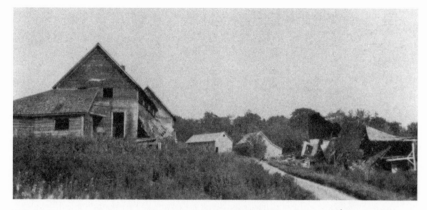

3.6 "Sylvania is another world," wrote Elin Anderson. The deserted village, once a thriving farming and lumbering center, had become " a bleak wilderness . . . this tomb of a village slowly falling into ruins." Sylvanians, content with the status quo, did not share Vermont Commission on Country Life officers' desire to develop their town into a tourist area. *Fifth Annual Report of the Eugenics Survey of Vermont*, 1931. Courtesy Special Collections Department, University of Vermont Library.

were abandoned, and the once-thriving industries of the town lay in ruins. Among the remnants of "first families" that remained, there was little hope expressed for renewal of the town. The Sylvanians seemed either content with the status quo or resigned to their subsistence way of life, their "substandard schools" and the "bleak and weather-beaten" wilderness their town had become. In Anderson's estimation, Sylvania was "a hopeful reminder of the good judgment shown by the people of the town to move when they have learned of more favorable opportunities elsewhere." Anderson's analysis of the human factor in Sylvania (Jamaica) complemented the recommendations of the VCCL Committee on Land Utilization, which found "exceptional opportunities for the development of land resources" for recreational uses and summer homes in such towns.[89]

Rural Vermont: Cultivating Vermont's Fitter Families

The committees of the VCCL completed their final reports in January 1931 and compiled their findings in *Rural Vermont: A Program for the Future*. Offered as a guide for rural planning based on scientific research, *Rural Vermont* was also a testimonial to the epic struggle of Vermonters to preserve the imagined America of the past. It was a plea for protection and support of the state's natural beauty and distinct historical heritage, which the enterprising participants of the commission sought to nurture and preserve. The "two hundred Vermonters" who had participated in the VCCL survey understood that their mission involved the conservation of the particular human stocks that had settled and created Vermont in the colonial days, along with their institutions and the monuments to their culture (old buildings, working farms, and attractive villages). Each committee produced a chapter in *Rural Vermont* that described Vermont's varied natural and human resources and gave recommendations for how local organizations, in collaboration with state government, could use the proposed "Program for the Future" as a guidebook or model plan for community renewal. Eugenics philosophy, whether consciously applied or not, was elaborated, diffused, and submerged within the reports of the various committees and frequently surfaced, though often in a sublimated form. Every chapter addressed the specific means by which the state could restore the land, culture, and values to the kind of people who had colonized the state and who were most deserving of the title "Vermonter."

Executive Director Henry C. Taylor's introduction to *Rural Vermont* described the VCCL in terms of human conservation: to maintain the fertility and quality of "one of the most reliable seedbeds of our national life," namely, the pioneer stocks who settled Vermont. Invoking the state motto, "Freedom and Unity," Taylor set the purpose and product of the enterprise within the paradigm of the ideal Vermonter: "While Vermonters are strongly individualistic—independent in thought and action—yet as a people, they are coherent and capable of working together. They live their own lives, knowing that others prize and choose a different course. They are a spirited people. They meet the challenge when obstacles stand in their pathway, but they do not let others mark the goals toward which they strive."[90]

In his sentimental chapter titled "Vermont," Justice Wendell P. Stafford celebrated the uniqueness of Vermont's landscape and culture, the special place Vermont held in the heart of every American who knew its beauty, its history, and its potential for future greatness. Excluded from Stafford's ode to Vermonters and his history of the state was the slightest recognition that the state was inhabited by French Canadian settlers or Indians prior to its colonization by New Englanders. "Native American" in *Rural Vermont* referred to English colonial settlers, their descendants, and White immigrants who had assumed the identity of "Yankee." French Canadians were cast as immigrants, whose presence postdated the founding of the state. Indians were not mentioned at all, implicitly sustaining the fiction that they had abandoned Vermont prior to statehood. "The people who first settled Vermont," according to the Committee on the Human Factor, "in the middle and latter part of the eighteenth century, were chiefly of English origin." They constituted the more rugged, adventuresome, and independent stocks from southern New

England "who were admirably fitted to make homes for themselves in the dense wilderness which then covered the state."[91]

Using this particular version of Vermont history as a point of departure, the report of the Committee on the Human Factor, "The People," described the population trends that had ensued over the next century and a half. Restoration of the fine innate qualities of the Vermont people would become a matter of population management. The Committee on the Human Factor resorted to maps and statistics to depict the (dysgenic) population trends that required attention. Seven maps sprinkled with dots illustrated the redistribution of Vermonters in the state and across the nation. A map of "Native Vermonters" listed in *Who's Who in America* reminded readers of Vermont's contribution of its native daughters and sons to the leadership of America. Maps also depicted the gradual concentration of younger Vermonters in urban centers at the expense of certain rural areas, particularly those along the backbone of the Green Mountains. The maps substantiated the long-held anxieties over the loss of excellent germplasm from rural Vermont and restated the urgency for its replenishment.

The Committee on the Human Factor recommended a program of "positive eugenics." Vermonters should be encouraged to study their family pedigrees to instill pride in the accomplishments of their "ancestral stock" and foster an awareness of the importance of good breeding. Education in the principles of eugenics, heredity, and population science in schools, public lectures and library resources, along with genealogical study, would nurture a general public sensitivity to ancestry and wise mate selection. Every "normal" couple in Vermont should view it as their patriotic duty to have sufficient children to replenish "the good old Vermont stock." Finally, local and state leaders should support programs that improve the quality of life for such wholesome Vermont families and relieve any financial burdens or social obstacles contributing to the rural exodus of "native stock."[92]

The Subcommittee on the Care of the Handicapped reported the needs of Vermont's social problem group in the chapter titled "The Care of the Handicapped." Henceforth, towns should work in close partnership with the state Department of Public Welfare to standardize the delivery of poor relief and psychiatric services. Rural towns should enlist the expertise of professionals in the diagnosis, supervision, and management of the feebleminded, insane, poor, and delinquent persons in their communities. The state should improve services to the poor by closing poorhouses and poor farms and by enlarging the Department of Public Welfare's role in supervising town overseers of the poor, establishing district welfare units, and standardizing and coordinating procedures for care of dependent Vermonters. In the interest of children, the Department of Public Welfare should develop parent education programs and conduct family casework. Traveling psychiatric clinics, more parole and probation officers, and development of case files on juvenile offenders for use by juvenile court judges would help to keep the problem of delinquency in abeyance. The Children's Charter was cited in support of district welfare offices, which called for "full time public welfare service for the relief, aid, and guidance of children in special need due to poverty, misfortune, or behavior difficulties, and for the protection of children from abuse, neglect, exploitation, or moral hazard."[93]

With the exception of the proposal for district welfare offices and the authority drawn from the 1930 White House Conference on Child Health and Protection, the new program for Vermont's handicapped appears to be simply a repackaged version of the fifteen-year-old agenda of Vermont's progressive coalition, which had begun with K. R. B. Flint's *Poor Relief in Vermont* (1916) and the Children's Aid Society's multifaceted project to preserve wholesome family groups. The fact that half of the committee consisted of Eugenics Survey advisory committee members, all of whom were also active members of the Vermont Conference of Social Work, explains the obvious continuity in theme and substance. But the old program in the new package had also undergone a transmutation, a subtle one of both crucial historical importance and tragic irony. The key element was this: communities in the future would assume the responsibility for their dependent, delinquent, and handicapped citizens, and every effort would be made to return those in state institutions to their families and integrate them as fully as possible into community life.

The White House conference had condemned social workers' past practice of breaking up families for "reasons of poverty alone." The Subcommittee on the Care of the Handicapped, conveniently forgetting the events of Children's Year and the early 1920s, transferred the blame for broken families to the overseers of the poor and to the state for its failure to provide adequate Mothers' Aid allowances. "All too frequently the home is needlessly broken up and children placed in institutions or foster homes," they reported. Welfare Commissioner Dyer sidestepped his department's previous complicity in the process by attributing the "broken health" and undernourishment of many children sent to institutions to poormasters' practice of placing destitute mothers in the poorhouse and their children in unsuitable foster homes. "Public sentiment in the towns where this may be the practice," he argued, "should be aroused to the extent that such methods be stopped for they are barbarous and relics of the slavery days that have no place in our beloved State of Vermont." Ironically, with the help of the Department of Charities and Probation and the Vermont Children's Aid Society, the "barbarous" practice of breaking up families and placing them in institutions or foster care had provided the source material for three years of eugenics investigations, which this committee cited only in a few footnotes. Yet in 1931, as in 1921, the sanction against breaking up families applied to "all family homes worthy of the name home" and excepted families with "unfit mothers."[94]

In the new program for the handicapped, the state would be expected to provide sufficient appropriations to establish district welfare offices and traveling psychiatric clinics, staffed by professional social workers, and also to provide sufficient poor relief to dependent mothers so that they might have a decent standard of living and a suitable home for their children. Many mentally and physically handicapped persons, they argued, could be successfully integrated into their home communities with appropriate supervision. Early diagnosis of mental and physical handicaps in children, followed by careful management of individual cases, would prevent later manifestations of delinquency and developmental disabilities.

Despite its expressed concern for the unresolved problems of Vermont's feebleminded population, the Subcommittee on the Care of the Handicapped made no mention of eugenics. Perkins added his own thoughts on the "Eugenic Aspects" in a special addendum to the report. Once again he summarized the results of the family studies and provided tables of "defects" of the fifty-five families and the public expense of ten of them from earlier annual reports. While arguing for "prevention of further defectiveness" through "strict enforcement of our laws governing marriage of defectives and such other measures as are calculated to check the multiplication of the unfit," Perkins set the old data in the new model of eugenic solutions through community cooperation: "The immediate need is to *lessen the distress of body or of mind* in those about us. Common humanity calls for that. . . . No hamlet is so small as to be exempt and every state and town has problems of its own *concerning its unfortunate, its underprivileged, its handicapped. . . .* How can a community, after caring to the best of its abilities for those who suffer from devastating ills, proceed to *govern itself* in such a way as to better its chances for the future?"[95] (emphasis mine)

Perkins made negative eugenics a matter of community responsibility, which the progressive towns would adopt as expressions of humanitarianism, civic responsibility, and perspicacity. He defined welfare problems in terms of accidents of birth whose solution lay in "preventing future mishaps." The rewards lay in the future and in the direct relation between positive and negative eugenics: "There will be a larger proportion of the people who will enjoy the richer life that is made possible by sound minds in healthy bodies, and our children's children will be less hampered by the social and economic drag of avoidable low grade Vermonters." Professional experts could offer knowledge and suggestions, but in the end Vermonters who embraced "Coming Vermont" ultimately would decide how to use this knowledge for themselves.[96]

The eugenics message emerged in other contexts in *Rural Vermont*, though more implicitly and perhaps unconsciously. The Committee on Education Facilities for Rural People, for example, recommended an orientation course on "the economic and social problems in the typical Vermont community" for graduates of normal schools as a component of ongoing teacher training. In 1932, eugenics, taught by Elin Anderson of the Zoology Department, was recommended for education majors in the UVM bulletin. The Committee on Education Facilities called for intensive collaboration between the Department of Education and the Department of Public Welfare to establish procedures for examining schoolchildren for signs of deficiency, retardation, and emotional disturbance and to develop a centralized census of such children.[97]

The report of the Committee on Religious Forces is especially interesting in light of its relevance to the religious controversies over eugenics that crystallized in 1930 with the encyclical *Casti Connubi (On Christian Marriage)* issued by Pope Pius XI. The pope unequivocally condemned eugenics, especially sterilization, matrimony based on heredity, and all other forms of family planning that interfered with the body's natural functions. Governor Weeks, chairman of the commission and a tacit supporter of eugenics, chaired the Committee on Religious Forces and was certainly aware of Catholic opposition to modern secular interventions in marriage and family life. While family planning was never an explicit theme in the country life movement, the vitality and influence of the Protestant country church as a social center in rural communities had always been a key component.[98] In Vermont, latent religious tension between Protestants and Catholic minorities presented an important obstacle to community solidarity. To confront the issue, the Committee on Religious Forces admitted that religious diversity, while potentially enriching community life, frequently made assimilation of Catholic, foreign immigrants into predominantly Protestant towns more difficult. They acknowledged the fact that Catholicism predated Protestant settlement, but because it was practiced in temporary French military encampments, they attributed the apparent Catholic intrusion into Protestant Vermont to more recent French and Irish immigration. French Canadians, who had a different language as well, presented a particular challenge to town unity. The map displaying the intermingling of Protestant churches, cooperative ministries, and Catholic churches and missions throughout the state emphasized the imperative for interfaith cooperation in community building. The solution, of course, was to encourage Vermonters of all faiths to join nonsectarian organizations in order to bridge religious barriers. French Canadian Catholics who had done so, such as the farmers in Cornwall, were generally respected.[99]

The Committee on Religious Forces offered the deistic tradition of the founding fathers and the ecumenical movement of the nineteenth century as a model to transcend religious exclusiveness in Vermont towns. Vermonters, they contended, had rejected Protestant evangelism as unsuited to their thirst for intellectual freedom, their belief in religious tolerance, and their aversion to demagoguery. Tolerance of religious freedom and subordination of religious dogmas to the common good would presumably enhance individual opportunities for self-realization. By offering this particular Protestant ethic as a measure of moral superiority, the Committee on Religious Forces reasserted their authority over religious matters in Vermont. Their position also provided an unstated admonition to Catholic priests who reputedly discouraged their parishioners from fraternizing with Protestants.[100]

Religious worship and education, however, presented practical difficulties. At best, the committee could only patronize Catholics by citing the many contributions of their schools, hospitals, and missions throughout the history of the state. It recommended a renewed affirmation of each church's efforts in the religious education of its youth to encourage leadership and high moral standards: "We are convinced that the future of our state and the very question of a livable social order depend upon the development of inner controls of conduct and the adequate preparation of youth for life in this changing world." To many Protestants in the 1930s (and to virtually all eugenicists), "inner controls" included restricting family size to the number of children that parents could support at least through high school and ideally through college. Championing tolerance and parents' obligation to prepare children for the modern world amounted to a veiled rebuttal of the pope's contention that the "family is more sacred than the state and that men are begotten not for the earth but for Heaven and eternity." The Catholic catechism was explicit on the obligations of married couples to have as many children as God gave them the ability to produce. Observant Catholics in Vermont in 1931 may have found their procreative choices more closely scrutinized in the confessional as well as by their Protestant neighbors. Considering Governor Weeks's support of the 1931 sterilization law, Catholic leaders probably found *Rural Vermont*'s report on religious forces patronizing, if not one more attempt to undermine Catholic teaching on the sacrament of marriage.[101]

Rural Vermont concludes with the report of the Committee on the Conservation of Vermont Traditions and Ideals, made up of Vermont writers and intellectuals who celebrated the exceptional beauty of Vermont and the unique character of Vermonters. They inaugurated a campaign to collect, preserve, and display all the cultural monuments to Vermont's heroic history. The VCCL would plan and support historic preservation of Vermont architecture, distribute works on Vermont history, literature, and biography to schools and libraries, and rejuvenate traditional Vermont folk music, arts, and crafts. Authors Dorothy Canfield Fisher and Sara Cleghorn, the committee's two most famous members, enhanced the status and visibility of the Vermont Country Life Commission. Cleghorn's pageant, "Coming Vermont," a special offering for the celebration of the publication of *Rural Vermont*, forecast a future generation of Vermonters rejoicing in a revival of the music, poetry, and traditions of their ancestors. Fisher, especially in later works, celebrated Vermonters as an unusual people whose history and way of life embodied independence, tolerance, and community spirit.[102]

Many historians and commentators on the Vermont Commission on Country Life have noted the implicit racism in *Rural Vermont* but have found its connection to eugenics elusive. Probably many, if not most, of the participants in the rural survey paid little attention to eugenics and used *Rural Vermont* as a forum to promote their own agendas and an opportunity to renew their commitment to the traditions of their state. But cultivating the "human factor" was the goal of nearly all committees; and those surveying Vermont's natural resources supported conservation and resource management policies conducive to the desired human development. The identity of Vermonters as a people unusually committed to their heritage, the preservation of their natural and cultural resources, and their continued quest of self-improvement provided the unifying (and tacitly eugenic) themes in *Rural Vermont*. Most important, as VCCL director H. C. Taylor contended, its central focus on the human factor made the Vermont commission unique among all country life programs in America. Taylor attributed this unique feature to Harry Perkins's inspiration from his work with the Eugenics Survey. Vermont Commissioner of Public Welfare William H. Dyer concurred with Taylor's assessment and congratulated Perkins on his success, predicting that "the work of the Eugenics Survey before many years will be one of the bright spots in the survey history of the State of Vermont, as I feel the matters that are being investigated and proven will be of inestimable value in the years to come."[103]

To Harry Perkins, *Rural Vermont* was the finest expression of a eugenics program and the fulfillment of his vision of population improvement through positive and negative eugenics, one in direct relation to the other. The "eugenic family," or "fitter family," was the ideal Vermont family, the "wholesome family" that the Vermont Children's Aid Society had made it their mission to protect and that the VCCL's demographic studies had found to dominate the state. With improvements in rural services, an invigoration of cultural and civic life, and a reduction in the burden of poor relief and care of the handicapped, rural towns in Vermont had every promise of attracting and sustaining the quality of family life required to restore Vermont to its place of honor as the seedbed of American leadership. The "other Vermont," its dysgenic element, could be managed through the progressive cooperation of schools, social agencies, and communities working in conjunction with the state Department of Public Welfare. Elin Anderson had predicted that dysgenic communities like "Sylvania" would probably die a natural death, as its residents, lacking the spirit of "rustic renewal," were encouraged to move to more progressive communities. These relocated Vermonters would either be stimulated to a higher level of achievement or would receive special assistance from the Department of Public Welfare and associated agencies. Their lands could revert to the public domain or be converted to tourist, recreation, or forestry services. Vermonters, through the comprehensive rural survey, had realized their biological and cultural worth and could, through their own combined efforts, produce a eugenics program second to none in the nation.

This was precisely the message Perkins delivered to the American and international eugenics community in the 1930s through articles in their periodicals, reviews, and papers delivered at eugenics conferences. Charles Davenport may have been the high priest of American eugenics, but Perkins had proved him wrong about the decline in the quality of Vermonters and about the insignificance of Perkins's small enterprise. With no tangible support from either Cold Spring Harbor or the American Eugenics Society, Perkins had provided the vision and leadership for a cooperative, community-based program of human self-improvement, based on a statewide scientific study of problems and solutions. When Perkins discussed *Rural Vermont* in national forums, he made a virtue of Vermont's smallness and perceived insignificance. With only "modest" resources and a "modest" but highly motivated and exceptionally capable group of volunteers and professionals, Vermonters had built a program of human improvement on the finest traditions of American democracy.[104]

"Voluntary" Sterilization in Vermont

In January 1931, as the reports for *Rural Vermont* were being completed, a new campaign for sterilization was mounted. "An Act for Human Betterment by Voluntary Sterilization" was closely aligned in language and purpose with the more benevolent tenor of the VCCL. The 1931 effort was led by members of the Committee on the Care of the Handicapped, who promoted voluntary sterilization as part of the new agenda to return institutionalized persons to their families and communities. Dr. E. A. Stanley, superintendent of the Waterbury State Hospital, and Dr. Truman Allen, superintendent of Brandon Training School, provided the public with a knowledge of expert opinion. They downplayed the role of heredity (inherited defects) and targeted instead the problem of the "social unfitness" of mentally disabled persons to raise children. A rhetoric of freedom and new opportunities for handicapped persons replaced the old "menace of the feebleminded," a reflection of the new consensus in institutional psychiatry.[105]

Possibly Perkins's role in the renewed effort was to keep the "overzealous proponents" of 1927 out of the way and perhaps to maintain a low profile himself. The American Eugenics Society had contacted Perkins in December 1930, urging him to propagandize on behalf of sterilization and activate his "Vermont State Committee." Perkins requested a postponement of their involvement, as he already expected a forthcoming legislative campaign on behalf of legalized sterilization. He confessed, with an air of apology, that he did not know such a state committee existed, and could they please send him a list of its members? Perkins's lapse of memory was probably intentional. His feigned ignorance of a state committee that he had agreed to chair and had helped to organize three years ago was perhaps a polite refusal of the sort of help that he blamed for the failure of the 1927 campaign.[106]

Perkins testified on behalf of the bill before the Public Health Committees of the House and Senate, alongside Dr. Allen and Dr. Stanley. He collected all the *Burlington Free Press* articles on the sterilization bill in 1931 and saved them in a personal scrapbook, as private testimony to the influence and efficacy of his eugenics teaching. Coverage of the legislative debates and letters to the editor reveal the extent that the public discourse in 1931 had turned on the issues of advocacy of the freedom of handicapped persons and tolerance of their presence in society. Perkins and his colleagues had carefully laid these foundations after 1927. Opponents to sterilization generally argued from a conservative position: such measures were unnatural, a violation of God's plan, and would only encourage immorality. They worried that the release of sterilized "incompetents" into Vermont communities would encourage promiscuity. Vermont towns, some argued, would once again be plagued with paupers, thieves, and sex delinquents. Some took issue with the hereditarian assumptions implied in the bill, arguing that the problems of delinquency and dependency were more rooted in neglect of religion and the decadent trends in modern society than in heredity. Some questioned the competency or objectivity of country doctors or overseers of the poor who could put candidates forth for sterilization. Were they qualified to diagnose congenital mental disorders or could they be trusted not to abuse the law? One lonely skeptic raised the question of professional integrity in a poem loaded with biting irony, perhaps aimed at the Eugenics Survey's agenda. E. F. Johnstone's "Authority to Mutilate" suggested that the doctors would all too quickly abandon their ethics for profit, eagerly hunting down poor, unconventional, or unwitting Vermonters if the state gave approval:

> When a doctor wants a boat
> On the broad highways to float
>   He will find a place where sapheads congregate
> He will chase them to a shed
> And at fifty bucks a head
>   He will freeze his conscience out and mutilate.

L. R. Weston of Cambridge, Vermont, also lampooned the bill by recommending an amendment requiring ear tags for sterilized persons, like the ones used for tuberculosis-tested cattle, so that they could be recognized "and they would never need be humiliated a second time by a clinical examination."[107]

The advocates of sterilization took a progressive tone: they emphasized the benefits of surgery for patients, currently cruelly confined to institutions, who could otherwise marry and lead normal lives. Dr. Truman Allen guaranteed the safety of the operation, its noninterference with normal sexuality, and the legal safeguards of the law against hasty or prejudiced diagnoses. He minimized the significance of heredity, arguing that mentally handicapped persons made inadequate parents; they had a difficult time supporting themselves, and the burden of children was more than they could bear. Other proponents cited the rising costs of institutional care and compared the estimated number of mentally deficient persons in the country receiving or awaiting special care to the cost of their sterilization. Some associated the growing problems of child neglect and abandonment with the uninhibited procreation by mentally incompetent parents and argued on behalf of the rights of the unborn to be "equipped with a good mind and body" and competent parents. The constitutionality of the sterilization act was defended by Oliver Wendell Holmes's 1927 opinion, rendered in *Buck v. Bell*, and the successful passage of such laws in twenty-three other states.

Nowhere were heard the voices of those who would be most affected by the bill raised. The Gypsies and Pirates, the Doolittles and Maggie Simpsons, the women at the Rutland Reformatory, the persons on the Brandon waiting list were not included in the hearings, nor did they write letters to the editors of newspapers covering the debates. That the "problem" posed to Vermont communities by these persons was really a problem of definition or of manifest historical intolerance never surfaced in serious discussion of the law. The 1931 debates had become a battle for advocacy of those whose lives would be changed forever by the bill and whose interest each side claimed to protect.

The progressive forces ultimately won their campaign. In March 1931 the General Assembly passed "An Act for Human Betterment by Voluntary Sterilization" by a substantial margin despite vehement minority opposition; Governor Stanley Wilson signed the bill on March 31. While Perkins claimed credit for the successful passage of the sterilization law through his survey's studies and their publication, he persistently denied that implementation had ever been part of the survey's mission. The record suggests that the law passed on the condition that sterilizations would be permitted only upon the recommendation of physicians and with the informed consent of the patient.[108]

The Eugenics Survey archive does not document sterilizations resulting from the law, much to the frustration of those who hold Perkins and his field staff responsible for the coerced or unwitting sterilization of their relatives. Because legal sterilizations took place for the most part in institutional settings, the identities of persons sterilized under the law remain hidden in the confidential case files of the Department of Public Welfare. "Authorized personnel" had unrestricted access to the family records that the Eugenics Survey field staff had collected, collated, and meticulously cross-indexed, but whether they were used or their contents communicated informally within the small, cohesive network of social workers in Vermont remains a matter of speculation. Perkins's own recollection—that once the sterilization law was passed, the survey no longer was involved except through general eugenics education—is probably correct. In 1931 the survey focused on community enrichment and immigration questions, and Perkins's new interest in the birth control movement began to replace his fascination with sterilization. Only by an accident of history or negligence on the part of Perkins's successor did the confidential case files of the Eugenics Survey enter the public record so that we might understand the process by which particular Vermont families, in a single decade, became "notorious" and ultimately lost their connection with family, community, and their history—in short, their humanity.

Those who find this episode in Vermont history regrettable should think seriously about how the accumulation of evidence and the consensus of experts empowers assumptions. Repetition of the findings of trusted scientists, layered in ever more sophisticated studies and fortified by the *convergence* of empirical data from diverse fields on the same question, galvanizes public and professional opinion. Researchers, abandoning untenable opinions when they discover their error, habitually absolve themselves of the responsibility for the uses that others, inspired by their findings, may find for their work. Take, for example, the events of Children's Year (1918–1919), when dozens of families were dissolved in an effort to repair "broken little lives." Here was the first step: an intelligent, well-intentioned, and trusted group of professionals and public servants broke up a number of families and thus provided an experimental population for the study of social problems. Six years later, those families with records in state institutions were recycled through the investigations and interventions of the Vermont Children's Aid Society and the state Department of Charities and Probation, while their personal and private histories receded beneath charts, statistics, and an ever more benevolent rhetoric of concern for their welfare. The pedigree work of Harriett Abbott and Francis Conklin probably inspired the subsequent investigation and incarceration of relatives of the broken family. Expansion of their representation in state correctional facilities and the confidential records of welfare agencies fortified their "notoriety" within Vermont's intimate and cooperative circle of social reformers. Families who reunited and returned to their communities on conditional parole likely faced censure. With a record and a reputation, their chances of rejection and recidivism would be great. The simple fact that Harriett Abbott or other social workers appeared in town asking questions about the character, problems, and reputation of the family would have fueled prejudice, validated suspicions, and amplified neighbors' "selective noticing" of the problems of the broken family. For those who volunteered evidence against particular families, Perkins's pejorative representations might have alleviated any guilt the informants suffered on account of their gossip and helped to transform their resentment of the family into open hostility.

After 1931 greater cooperation of schools and communities with the Department of Public Welfare would strengthen public sensitivity to pathological behavior and mental deficiency, and "good parenting" would include acquiescence with the recommendations of experts in child psychology regarding accommodations for any handicapped children. While social workers promised to stop taking children from their parents for poverty alone, the damage had already been done. After a decade of repeated intervention and investigations of certain families, their fate would be decided by mental test results and proof of compliance with conditions of parole, not the prejudice or poverty that might have generated their problems. Eugenics theory was founded on a *perception* that social dysfunction was spreading, like a malignancy, through reproduction. Yet the reproduction of evidence by eugenicists and well-intentioned social reformers and its propagation throughout the professional literature of diverse fields and the public domain were probably more toxic to children and families than real or imaginary genes.

In 1931, Professor Perkins, who had built his scientific reputation on the misfortunes of others, stepped into the national limelight, and Vermonters celebrated their renewed identity and the dawning of a new future promised in *Rural Vermont*. An unknown number of other Vermonters, who stood in the shadows as their nearly forgotten histories began collecting dust in the Eugenics Survey files, were poised to sacrifice their parenthood for the presumed benefit of other people's children.

National Recognition, Crisis, and Reform, 1931–1939

We pay full price for the virtues our culture develops at any particular period. . . . The very ethnic and religious prejudices which still live in the community may be forged into the tools by which a demagogue can further divide the population and stultify human development.

—Elin Anderson, *We Americans*, 1937

It should be clearly recognized that the test of the calibre of our democracy will be judged according to the manner in which we treat our underprivileged groups, at the same time striving to improve our human stock.

**—Frederick C. Thorne, Medical Director,
Brandon Training School, 1946**

The Realization of a Dream, 1931–1933

In 1931, it appeared that the original goals of the Eugenics Survey of Vermont had been achieved. At Perkins's urging, the Eugenics Survey advisory committee agreed to devote its efforts over the next year to promoting *Rural*

Vermont throughout the state and supporting community efforts to implement its recommendations. The Eugenics Survey would take the initiative in
this effort through sponsoring adult education programs and public lectures,
leading round-table discussions and community study groups, and distribut-
ing relevant source material to clubs, schools, and libraries. Elin Anderson, as
the new assistant director of the Eugenics Survey, would become the driving
force behind this campaign.[1]

Harry Perkins, having succeeded his aging father as director of the University Museum in 1926, assumed new responsibilities and acquired a broader
visibility as the new Robert Hull Fleming Museum was completed in 1931.
The new facility, with its marble court and richly appointed reading rooms,
required new programs commensurate with its design and with its new status
as a monument to the natural and cultural history of the state. Perkins developed the museum into a new venue for Vermonters' cultural enrichment. No
longer a repository of curios, bird and animal specimens, and Indian artifacts
collected by his father, the new museum would be a center for education
through special programs and projects to stimulate Vermonters' appreciation
of their history. It became the repository of the Wilbur collection of Ver-
montiana; the center for the historic preservation of old buildings, directed
by Perkins and Herbert Congdon; and the film lending library for public
schools. (Fig. 4.1.)

While Vermont communities, with Anderson's guidance, collaborated to
create the eugenic future outlined in *Rural Vermont*, the national eugenics
movement was beginning to disintegrate into factions. Intellectual leaders in
science, medicine, and sociology questioned more openly the scientific validity of eugenics research and the legitimacy of exploiting dubious studies
on race and class differences to shape mental health programs and immi-
gation policy. To many socialists, eugenics had become tool to oppress the
lower classes and ethnic minorities. Opposition came from conservative and
religious groups as well. Catholics, especially, organized effective campaigns
to oppose sterilization laws in many states. The most pressing concern to
the American eugenics leadership, however, was a growing public apathy toward eugenics and a corresponding decline in financial support as the Depression diverted resources to more immediate needs. Disagreements among
the leaders of the movement festered privately, while publicly they maintained a show of unity. The growing tensions reached a climax in May 1931
and precipitated a crisis within the American Eugenics Society (AES). At
this juncture, Harry Perkins was invited into the national spotlight with his
unanimous election as vice president at the annual meeting of the AES on
May 25, 1931.[2]

When he accepted the nomination, Perkins had not been involved in the
inner circle of national eugenics and was unaware of the depth and severity of

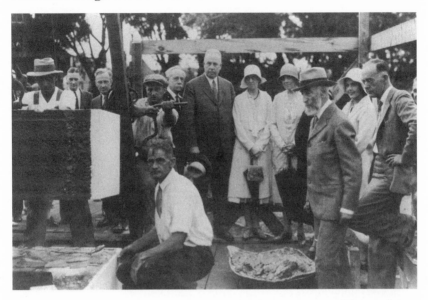

4.1 Professor Harry Perkins (*far right*) and his daughter Anne (*second from right*) look on as Dean George H. Perkins steps forward to lay the cornerstone for the Fleming Museum on 1 July 1930. UVM president Guy W. Bailey, a member of the Eugenics Survey advisory committee, is standing sixth from the left. From University of Vermont, *Vermont* (Winter 1985): 65. Courtesy Special Collections Department, University of Vermont Library.

its internal grievances. As such, he was the perfect "dark horse." Perkins's relations with the leaders in American eugenics had been polite and professional, even deferential. Charles Davenport and Arthur Estabrook, who served on the AES nominating committee, understood Perkins's serious commitment to eugenics and had always found him especially impressionable. Perkins's willingness to apply sociological methods and insights to eugenics appealed to the younger, more environmentally oriented faction in the AES, led by Frederick Osborn and Yale geographer Ellsworth Huntington. Frederick Osborn, a wealthy businessman and nephew of eugenicist-anthropologist Henry Fairfield Osborn, had taken up serious study of eugenics in 1928 and was keenly interested in social factors affecting population trends. Huntington must have appreciated Perkins's implementation of his suggestions in the human factor study for the Vermont Commission on Country Life (VCCL), and Osborn, who also served on the AES nominating committee, had known and admired Perkins's work for some time. Perkins's reputation as a scientist was not in dispute, his position on sterilization was moderate, and he had remained aloof, publicly at least, from the controversies over eugenics and race. Perkins, having shown himself responsive to persuasion by both factions, was an ideal compromise candidate, one who might help to dissipate the growing dissension within the national movement.[3]

For Perkins, this new office was a mixed blessing, presenting both serious practical problems and intriguing opportunities. To assume a position of leadership in the national movement would certainly bring his Vermont projects national visibility and would raise his own prestige within the state. On the other hand, as he immediately discovered, the AES was on the verge of collapse; election to its board of directors was a dubious honor. The society was $7,000 in debt, and creditors were threatening to bring legal action. After surveying the damage and concluding that the situation was hopeless, President-elect Clarence Campbell (also president of the Eugenics Research Association) immediately resigned and retreated to Cold Spring Harbor. Harry Laughlin, Albert Wiggam, and Judge Harry Olson quickly followed Campbell's lead, leaving Perkins alone on the stage without the star cast or the experience to perform the new role. Their sudden mass exodus was simply the culmination of a more gradual retiring of biologists from the organization, whose membership had once enhanced the prestige of the society and had attracted endowments before the onset of the Depression.[4]

Perkins, bewildered by it all, hesitated to relinquish the opportunity to take Campbell's place as president, despite the society's problems. He solicited the opinions of Campbell and Laughlin and of Paul Popenoe and Edwin Gosney from the West Coast branch, and he queried all parties involved in its problems. Perkins learned at the outset that most of the society's problems were the result of poor fiscal management, personality conflicts, and philosophical differences, especially on the issue of birth control. Moreover, he discovered that the important men in American eugenics respected his scientific reputation, his intelligence and his integrity and would support his efforts to salvage the foundering society. Finally, all accusing fingers pointed to the society's executive director, Leon Whitney, whose outspoken self-righteousness had alienated those who opposed his views and outraged creditors whose requests he ignored. Whitney's populist programs, like "fitter family" and sermon contests, had become the scapegoat for the society's fiscal problems. Perkins could see that what was needed was diplomacy, sensitivity to the political climate and potential sources of conflict, a commitment to cooperation, and a sincere effort to pay off the debts. His experience and talent in these areas had been successful in the past, and he met the challenge of the AES crisis years with the same style and dedication he had brought to eugenics work in Vermont.[5]

Over the next three years, the solvency, reputation, and the growing pains of the American eugenics movement occupied Perkins's time and energy. He mediated disputes, respected confidences, and sympathized with the grievances of those, like Leon Whitney, who felt misunderstood, slighted, or wronged. He stressed the importance of cooperation, solidarity, and prudence. He personally approached a number of foundations for grants and conducted a national membership campaign to help alleviate the debt and pay the back salaries of the office staff, which, he contended, was a moral obligation. During the Depression, his fund-raising efforts met with marginal success, although many former supporters, unable to make a donation, encouraged his efforts to promote eugenics. By 1932 the society had reduced its debt from $7,000 to $1,500, a fact that the next AES president, Ellsworth Huntington, attributed to Perkins's able leadership.[6]

If the AES was to survive at all, it had to establish its scientific credibility through formal alliances and joint publications with scientific organizations devoted to the study of population trends and human betterment. In the early 1930s, the Eugenics Research Association at Cold Spring Harbor still enjoyed the support of the Carnegie Institution of Washington, despite the criticism of its research by eminent scientists. Perkins, a self-described "inveterate merger," helped to negotiate a partnership of AES and the Eugenics Research Association, in which they would sponsor joint annual meetings and collaborate on the publication and distribution of *Eugenical News*. Perkins agreed to serve on the editorial board; it was also agreed that the articles on genetics and population science would dominate and that editorials on eugenics theory and public policy would appeal to reason, not politics or emotion. Frederick Osborn, who later convinced historians that he had almost single-handedly led the reform of the AES and its renunciation of the Cold Spring Harbor group, actually sat on the boards of both societies and assisted Perkins behind the scenes with this merger. Osborn nevertheless conceded that Perkins's "more thoughtful approach" helped to rehabilitate the AES at a critical juncture in the organization's history.[7]

Perkins facilitated mergers with other organizations—internally debated, privately negotiated, and carefully choreographed. Joint meetings or conferences served as a prelude to more formal connections in the form of interlocking directorships on executive boards, joint publications, and shared membership lists for promotional literature reflecting the mutual goals of each society. Because the AES could ill afford to alienate potential sponsors by attracting controversy, its officers wished to avoid involvement with groups known for populist or partisan agendas. Only after much deliberation and Perkins's urging, for example, did they agree to collaborate with the Birth Control League, the predecessor of Planned Parenthood. Most leaders in American eugenics held conservative views regarding the decriminalization of the distribution of contraceptives and birth control information and had refused to associate with the movement's leader, Margaret Sanger. Perkins, however, embraced birth control as a tool of eugenics with as much enthusiasm as he had favored eugenic sterilization in the decade earlier and privately encouraged his colleagues to offer their official support. Responses were mixed at first, but the partnership with the Birth Control League succeeded during Perkins's tenure. The Population Association of America and the American Statistical Association also responded to the AES overtures for joint conferences.[8]

To establish its credibility within the scientific and medical establishment the AES had to revise its philosophy in accordance with scientific criticism of its previous positions. The revision would require the society to acknowledge the complex causes of mental illness and retardation, distance itself from a rhetoric of exclusion and Anglo-Saxon superiority, and, in light of the economic depression, eliminate prosperity and social position as indicators of genetic superiority. The importance of a revision of Leon Whitney's *Eugenics Catechism* (1926) was recognized prior to Perkins's election to the board, and Huntington and Perkins worked intermittently over the next three years on a revised catechism. Perkins fully understood the problems with the society's literature from his own experience with it in Vermont with the 1927 sterilization campaign. And just prior to his election to the AES executive board, Perkins once again discovered the political liability of Leon Whitney's promotions. At Whitney's urging, Perkins had flirted with the immigration issue, using the AES Committee of Selective Immigration report as source material to produce a sample newsletter. His advisory committee vetoed the *Immigration and Eugenics* circular, which advocated stricter quotas on "racially inferior" immigrants. Asa Gifford had brought Perkins to a complete halt by warning him that "anything sent out by the Survey should be precise and scientifically acceptable. . . . This offering is neither—is the production of a *Propagandist!*" With these problems in mind, Perkins appreciated the need for a complete revision of the society's philosophy, but a society in debt could not launch any new projects. Hence, work on the revised catechism was largely neglected until 1933, when world and domestic developments gave urgency to a reformulated position.[9]

Perkins had more success using his national position to promote the Eugenics Survey of Vermont and the VCCL to counter popular images of Vermonters as naive and backward and to advertise their unique progressive program for rural eugenics. In the wake of his publicity, requests for the Eugenics Survey annual reports poured in during the early 1930s as favorable reviews of the rural survey engendered interest. Elin Anderson's migration study in the fifth annual report attracted the most attention, and Perkins seemed content to serve as her agent rather than her superior. While many of the requests came from scholars in rural sociology and agricultural studies, contemporaries understood the eugenic nature of the migration study. *Journal of Heredity* editor Robert C. Cook, for example, while criticizing the idea of "buying out" the marginal ruralist, praised the Eugenics Survey's rural survey as just the sort of eugenics research that was needed.[10]

The Third International Congress of Eugenics, held at the American Museum of Natural History in New York, August 21–23, 1932, offered another opportunity to promote *Rural Vermont*. Attendance at the third congress had dropped to seventy-four (over three hundred had met in 1921), yet the sixty-five papers presented showed the same diversity of scientific topics and eugenic commentaries that characterized the second congress and was attended by a number of notable biologists. Perkins gave a paper, "Contributory Factors in Eugenics in a Rural State," in which he presented the Vermont comprehensive rural survey as a eugenics project "built upon the fine traditions of the old state." Whereas VCCL director Henry C. Taylor had emphasized the grass-roots nature of the enterprise—a "study of Vermonters by Vermonters"—Perkins gave the eugenics congress a more candid view, stating that "the more intelligent and socially minded people of all walks of life in all parts of Vermont were gathered together" for the purpose of "clearing up some of the complications of conserving the good old Vermont stock in the rural parts."[11] Perkins emphasized the importance of environmental management in cultivating human resources: "No better eugenic program for any section of the country occurs to me than this: The improvement of living conditions, the encouragement of social and intellectual opportunities that will enrich the lives of the people making them aware of the trends of this modern age, including the trend of Eugenics, and affording them a richer environment in which to rear their children."

The Vermont solution to the rural degeneracy problem, Perkins concluded, was simply a matter of recognition that the superior genetic potential of the pioneer stocks had remained undeveloped without a suitable environment for its expression in the modern age: "A fine old pioneer stock deserves an environment commensurate with its quality and only in such an environment can the innate qualities of the people come to any worthy fruition. If their home surroundings are poor and life nothing better than a perpetual fight for the merest necessities, their native ambition may be so dampened as to make them indifferent to their future and that of their children."[12]

In his celebration of Vermont's new eugenic approach to the problem of rural decline, he neglected to mention that "clearing up complications" had involved negative eugenics measures applied to those Vermonters who purportedly had compromised the quality of life for Vermont's "elect." But anyone who visited the Eugenics Exhibit Hall at the congress would have understood. Perkins's exhibit displayed a fifteen-foot-long pedigree chart of one of Vermont's "complications": five generations of feeblemindedness, insanity, consanguinity, alcoholism, and men and women "living together, not legally married"—all traced from two boys at the Vermont Industrial School.[13]

"Is Eugenics Dead?"

Despite the efforts of eugenicists at the Third International Congress of Eugenics to establish the relevance of their research to current human affairs, public apathy to eugenics continued. The press more frequently portrayed eugenics in a negative light while publicizing the criticism of scientists who, for both professional and philosophical reasons, had abandoned the idea of directing the future course of human evolution. While the AES was struggling with its public image, its philosophy, and its ability to survive at all, President Perkins was called on to evaluate the progress of American eugenics. In its April 1933 issue, the *Journal of Heredity* published a forum on the question "Is Eugenics Dead?" A. W. Forbes, a wealthy businessman with a long-standing interest in positive eugenics, was concerned about the "moribund condition" of eugenics in America and suggested the discussion. He called on recognized leaders in American eugenics to provide an honest and reasoned assessment of the goals, accomplishments, scientific merit, and future of eugenics. Editor Robert C. Cook prefaced the forum with the American Genetics Society's policy to avoid "official axes to grind" and provide "accurate and unbiased information, not embarrassed by adherence to any particular 'program.'"[14]

The responses to Forbes's challenge revealed the philosophical tensions within the American eugenics movement, and despite Cook's warning, official axes were ground. Leon Whitney, for example, attributed the lack of progress in eugenics to insufficient funding, caused in part by the Depression but also by the failure of wealthy men like Forbes to recognize the value of programs directed toward changing popular opinion, the engine of social change. Michigan State College geneticist H. R. Hunt invoked the scientific progress argument, explaining how human genetics was in fact undergoing a revolutionary transformation. The "new eugenics" of the 1930s promised far more than the original highly politicized programs, whose oversimplification of the complexities of human heredity were a great embarrassment to the majority of researchers seeking *unbiased* knowledge of human heredity. Naturally, more funding of research in human heredity was needed.[15]

Clarence Campbell, as president of the Eugenics Research Association, presented a vehement defense of orthodox, hereditarian-based eugenics, attributing its lack of progress to the unwillingness of Americans to apply its findings. Given to immediate gratification of individual interests—and misguided by sociologists who refused to recognize that race betterment de-

pended on *biological* selection (not simply an improvement of living conditions)—Americans were too hesitant to strengthen or vigorously implement
immigration restrictions, antimiscegenation laws, and sterilization of the "biologically unfit." American couples, Campbell complained, were more interested in marital bliss than their patriotic obligation to channel their sexuality
into eugenic reproduction. Campbell used the term "race" or "racial" more
than twenty times in his defense of eugenics and forecast that America would
"deteriorate in its racial quality" and be "superseded in the domination and
unchallenged tenure of its territory . . . by a race of greater fertility, of greater
aggressive temperament, and of greater racial cohesion and integration."[16]

Perkins's contribution, an essay titled "Make Haste Slowly," differed from
the others in two important ways. First, he admitted the need for American
eugenicists to reconsider their program rather than defend its shortcomings.
Second, he appealed to the hopes of Americans rather than to their anxieties
and fears. There had been too much negativity in American eugenics, and he
had learned from experience just how counterproductive appeals to hate and
fear had been in his own promotion of eugenics in Vermont. The American
public, Perkins conceded, should not be expected to be very patient with a
movement that, by its definition, is vague and uncertain during a world
depression when all facets of life are uncertain. At such times a "judicious
combination of zeal and conservatism" was needed.[17] Once again Perkins
dispensed with the sterilization controversy by condemning it to history.
The "noisy propaganda" of the early eugenics movement, he explained, had
served its purpose of awakening the American public to the need for managing reproduction and creating an awareness of the dysgenic or eugenic influence of various home and social environments. But the passage of sterilization laws, he explained, had been misconceived as a total solution to human
betterment. The important effects of the eugenics movement, he argued,
were quietly and invisibly but more constructively at work. A sound eugenics
program would ultimately rest on public education in the principles of genetics and the role of environmental influences—social, cultural, and physical—
in the achievement of human potential. Biology and family life education
would cultivate an awareness of the social implications of reproductive behavior and foster a eugenic consciousness. Research into how families could
be made more effective, in size and quality, combined with a study of demographic trends, represented the more enlightened, if less dramatic, approach
to eugenics. These new trends, Perkins prophesied, would gradually replace
the eugenics of the past decade.[18]

Perkins never mentioned the projects of the Eugenics Survey of Vermont
in "Make Haste Slowly," but the "new trends" that he believed would replace
the old were already underway in Vermont—activities that Perkins had reported to the Eugenics Survey advisory committee the week prior to Cook's

request for a defense of eugenics. In the first year of the VCCL educational campaign, Elin Anderson gave over forty public lectures around the state, organized study groups in three rural towns to conduct local surveys, and began a weekly class on the care of the handicapped in a women's club in Burlington. She was currently teaching the eugenics course in the University of Vermont Zoology Department, which Perkins had delegated to her the year before. While Perkins wrote "Make Haste Slowly," Anderson was organizing a series of seminars, "Helping People in Need," through the Vermont Conference of Social Work to enable volunteers to consult with professional social workers.

Professor Perkins had contributed to the eugenics education campaign in other ways. He had developed a series of children's programs at the Fleming Museum, including a Fingerprint Club, which would cultivate biological and hereditary self-awareness. In his heredity course, Perkins instilled an appreciation of human heredity through student projects on identical twins inspired by H. H. Newman's studies and recent articles on twins in the *Journal of Heredity*. From his combined interests in the adoption program of the Vermont Children's Aid Society and twin studies, he had started an investigation of the effect of adoption on the ability of childless couples to conceive their own children. If adoption stimulated fertility, he reasoned, then it was eugenic, for it would enhance the fecundity of parents with a demonstrated capacity for nurturance and the ability to provide suitable homes for children. As executive vice president of the VCCL, Perkins promoted *Rural Vermont* in a radio series and led a discussion at the state teachers convention on the integration of heredity, eugenics, and sex education into the high school biology curriculum. For Harry Perkins these projects exemplified the more invisible and constructive eugenics of the future.[19]

The Eugenics Survey's most important project, of the sort that Perkins expected would replace the old eugenics, was a study of ethnic relations in Burlington and the influence of ethnic diversity on social factors operating in the city. The survey had never fully explored race or ethnicity as a variable in Vermont's "human factor" after Perkins had tabled the French Canadian issue in 1929. Since that time the Eugenics Survey library had acquired recent studies on assimilation of immigrants that provided different models to explore the eugenic significance of ethnic diversity. "Racial" differences— whether rooted in heredity, culture, or a combination of the two—were to Perkins the most obvious products of human evolution, and no eugenics program would be complete without a study of them. In 1932, Perkins announced that the survey would conduct a preliminary study of national ratios, birthrates, and factors influencing assimilation of immigrants in a single community, Burlington. Perkins granted Elin Anderson, whose diplomacy, intuition, and scholarship far exceeded his own, full autonomy over the project.

Anderson decided to explore the French Canadian question in a more comprehensive format: the study of ethnic relations as obstacles to community cohesiveness and individual self-realization.

Bessie Bloom Wessel's *Ethnic Survey of Woonsocket, Rhode Island* (1931) and Christine Avghi Galitzi's *Study of Assimilation among Roumanians in the United States* (1929) provided initial inspiration for Anderson; both had become important sources in the Eugenics Survey library collection of American "melting pot" studies. Wessel had studied the social obstacles to cultural and biological fusion, though intermarriage, of Woonsocket's immigrant communities. Like Vermont, Woonsocket had a large French Canadian (or Franco-American) population and also had endured friction between French and Irish factions of the Catholic community. Wessel had selected that city to fill the void in research on French Canadian immigrants. Christine Galitzi, herself a member of a Roumanian immigrant community in Chicago, investigated the sociological and cultural influences on Roumanian immigrants and their descendants as they adapted to American life. Her study challenged Americanization theories that measured the progress and adaptation of immigrants in terms of their adoption of "American" ideas, values, and lifestyles, which, she felt, "endorsed without reservation the 'Nordic Myth' as an unchallenged scientific truth that claims that Anglo-Saxon culture is the only one suitable to Americans."[20]

Burlington, however, was more like Robert S. and Helen Merrell Lynd's "Middletown" (Muncie, Indiana), whose biography and sociology had become the scholarly version of Sinclair Lewis's *Main Street*. The Lynds' *Middletown: A Study in American Culture* (1929) provided Anderson with a somewhat different model for her study of Burlington. The Lynds analyzed social and cultural factors that became reinforced through economic stratification and emphasized the role of attitudes as sociological forces. The Lynds' interviews of Middletown citizens' attitudes toward one another and to the social and economic pressures within the community provided Anderson with a model for investigating ethnic tensions. The Lynds' research for their second volume, *Middletown in Transition: A Study in Cultural Conflicts* (1937), paralleled Anderson's ethnic study of Burlington, and Robert Lynd became one of Anderson's key consultants for her project.[21]

In 1932, Anderson's eugenics class launched the ethnic study with a house-to-house canvas of the entire city of Burlington to establish the national derivation of the city's twenty-three thousand inhabitants and to determine their geographic distribution within its neighborhoods. With the help of her students, Anderson constructed a large spot map locating the homes of first- and second-generation Irish, Italian, French Canadian, Jewish, and German residents and "Old Americans." From these data a representative sample would be drawn for sociological analysis and interviews, in the manner of the

Lynds' studies of Middletown. But unlike the Lynds, Anderson encouraged the full knowledge and participation of the community in her research. Recognizing the importance of understanding the immigrants' experience from their point of view, Anderson hired six women, recognized members of each ethnic group in the study, to act as liaisons between their communities and the survey and to assist her in conducting the interviews and interpreting the information.

In the spring of 1933, Anderson had converted the Eugenics Survey office into a center for round-table discussions on such topics as the "Cause and Cure of War" and multiethnic study groups on "racial and cultural fusion." Just prior to Perkins's writing of "Make Haste Slowly," he had notified his advisory committee of Anderson's plans to survey the attitudes of old American stock, French Canadians, and other ethnic groups toward each other and toward interracial mingling. Her findings, he anticipated, would provide the information to consider the "eugenical significance of the American melting pot as found operating in Vermont."[22]

The progress of eugenics in Vermont, as Perkins now understood it, looked different from the visions of eugenics described by Clarence Campbell, Leon Whitney, and the others in the April 1933 forum "Is Eugenics Dead?" American eugenics was clearly at a crossroads but by no means dead. The future of eugenics, as described by each of these leaders in American eugenics, charted the course each would take as the German experiment in eugenics moved to center stage and changed forever the meaning of eugenics.

Eugenics in the New Germany and American Responses

In January 1933 the Nazis assumed power in Germany as Hitler was sworn in as chancellor. On April 1, 1933, the Nazi regime decreed the anti-Jewish boycott of Jewish-owned businesses and passed the Enabling Act, which established restrictive quotas for Jews serving in government positions, professions, and universities. These measures began the formal, government-sanctioned process of exclusion, public humiliation, and persecution of German Jews and triggered the first wave of Jewish refugees seeking asylum from the Nazi policies against groups they defined as alien. While political dissidents, Communists, Jehovah's Witnesses, and Catholics were persecuted in the Third Reich, Nazi "race hygiene" measures targeted other groups: those defined as biologically inferior by Aryan race theorists (Jews and Gypsies) and persons diagnosed as genetically diseased—the handicapped and "asocials" (homosexuals, sex offenders, criminals).

As part of its race hygiene program, the German government enacted a sterilization law in July 1933. "The Law for the Control of Hereditarily Diseased Offspring" established procedures for the compulsory sterilization of the mentally retarded, epileptics, criminals, the insane, and those having serious or disfiguring physical handicaps. The new program coordinated and deployed existing administrative bureaucracies and medical institutions to locate, identify, register, and surgically sterilize persons who displayed presumed hereditary defects. German eugenics was not a Nazi invention; the rationale, procedures, and medical and psychiatric research institutions for such a program had developed concurrently with the American and British research. The Nazi legislation, however, removed legal impediments to sterilization that had existed in the Weimar Republic and framed its purpose in terms of an urgent fight for survival of the German nation and the "Aryan race." German eugenicists and anthropologists who had opposed the theory of Nordic superiority, including some Jewish scientists, lost their positions in German universities. The familiar eugenic themes—economic burdens on the hardworking middle class, the rising costs of institutional care for the insane and feebleminded, and the failure of traditional therapy to reverse the rising tide of degeneracy—had resounded in German medicine and eugenics for three decades. Yet the loss of American loans due to the Depression gave urgency to economic arguments of the necessity to sterilize so-called useless eaters who were blamed for draining the resources of Germany's struggling middle class. The sterilization law went into effect on January 1, 1934, when an estimated four hundred thousand cases went before Hereditary Courts.[23]

If 1929–1933 had been a period of confusion, controversy, and review of eugenics in theory and practice, the Nazi experiment crystallized tensions over eugenics in science, medicine, and politics throughout the world. Discussion over the future of eugenics was no longer a matter of speculation; Germany had made it a matter of fact. From 1934 on, the application of human genetics in public health policy became linked to world politics. The political nature of German eugenics was reinforced, as many political dissidents, Communists, and nonconformists fell into the categories of mentally incompetent, incurable, and alien, and found themselves in penal and mental institutions as race hygiene policies were implemented. The diverse responses of American and British eugenicists (and geneticists) to these developments would further amplify public awareness of the political nature of the enterprise and force academic debates over the validity of its biological assumptions into the open.[24]

After World War II the Nazi radicalization of eugenics into genocide would demonstrate the potential for evil in eugenics ideology and would make prophets of its early critics, but the implications of the German sterilization program were not so obvious in 1934. Some found the German program enviable; campaigns for sterilization laws were launched in the United States and many nations abroad, including the Scandinavian countries, the Baltic states, Japan, and the Netherlands. Opponents of eugenics and sterilization, particularly Catholics, used Nazi experiments to portray sterilization as an instrument of tyranny, which exemplified all that was undemocratic in the eugenics movement. In 1934, Paul Popenoe of the Human Betterment Foundation in California believed that the German law was "well-drawn" but noted that its success "depends largely on its being administered conservatively, intelligently, and sympathetically."[25]

While the world anticipated and debated the significance of the new German sterilization program, Harry Perkins was busy writing letters to generate funds to retire the debts of the AES. Henry H. Goddard's response to Perkins's fund-raising efforts illustrates the mixed emotions the German program evoked:

> Why not drop the whole works? . . . We have carried on for several years and what have we accomplished? It was good fun as long as we could afford it, but now it is a different matter.
>
> If Hitler succeeds in his wholesale sterilization, it will be a demonstration that will carry eugenics farther than a hundred Eugenics Societies could. If he makes a fiasco of it, it will set the movement back where a hundred eugenic societies can never resurrect it.[26]

Goddard's prophetic letter, routinely cited as evidence of Perkins's pro-Nazi sentiments, speaks to our time but reveals nothing of Perkins's beliefs or the dilemma he faced in 1934. Goddard's cavalier attitude is interesting in light of his own leadership in American eugenics and the spectacular "fiasco" *he* had made of it in Ohio in the 1920s, in his failed attempt to create a state eugenics program through the Ohio Bureau of Juvenile Research. As a psychology professor at Ohio State University, Goddard, like Perkins and other eugenicists, had admitted the error of overemphasizing heredity at the expense of environmental factors in his early work on feeblemindedness.[27]

In reply to Goddard's letter, Perkins defended the American effort: "This very matter of the results of Hitler's program of wholesale sterilization appeals to me and to several of the members of our Advisory Council as being one of the most cogent reasons for carrying on." Perkins enclosed reprints of the forum "Is Eugenics Dead?" in the *Journal of Heredity* and referred Goddard to his own response, "Make Haste Slowly," which had reduced the early sterilization campaigns to a misunderstood panacea based on noisy propaganda.[28] Perkins and his colleague Ellsworth Huntington had, in fact, been "carrying on" by distancing the AES from organizations that had promoted views of Nordic racial superiority. The previous June, Perkins and Huntington had decided that the revision of the old eugenics "catechism" could no longer be postponed. Perkins had urged the publication of a pamphlet that could be produced sooner and be more widely distributed than the book Huntington had in mind.[29]

Perkins's problems with the future of eugenics or Hitler's program were not Goddard's. Perkins's concerns were more immediate and personal. In Vermont, Perkins had failed to persuade Shirley Farr to continue funding the Eugenics Survey; she had requested a release from her earlier commitments, wishing to consolidate her philanthropies as her health was failing. Perkins had tried without success to secure Elin Anderson a fellowship at Yale or a position with the Human Betterment Foundation in California.[30] In September, Harry's father, George Henry Perkins, died suddenly at the age of eighty-nine. By December, Harry Perkins's health failed as well, and his doctor advised him to take a rest. On December 31, the eve of the launching of the German sterilization program, Leon Whitney, still acting ostensibly as executive secretary of the AES, went out of control. He boasted to Perkins that the national press coverage of his views on the German sterilization program had elicited a publisher's request for a seventy-thousand-word book on the subject, which he had completed "in just two weeks."[31] Perkins had just spent the past year pleading with friends in Vermont and potential donors across America to help pay off the debts resulting in part from Whitney's prior indiscretions; he had generated only $78 and a snide response from Goddard. All efforts Perkins had made on behalf of the AES—financially, administratively, and philosophically—had failed.

Certainly discouraged, Perkins was probably dreading the fallout from Whitney's latest performance, especially in Vermont. Elin Anderson and her staff at the Eugenics Survey office had completed preliminary interviews of leaders in Burlington's various ethnic communities and were developing a questionnaire to survey large segments of Burlington's population concerning their experiences with ethnic intermingling and racial prejudices in the community. Anderson found the Germans to be especially reticent; many suspected that the ethnic survey was a cover for preparation for another war. Her Jewish informants were quite candid on the problem of anti-Semitism as an obstacle to their own participation in social and civic life. One Jewish man confided his opinion that demagogues, in trying to unite Protestants and Catholics, often used Jews as the common enemy. Another Jewish informant noted that eugenicists had hurt themselves by limiting their efforts to proving the superiority of the Nordic race and refusing to see the value of other peoples. Anderson's interviews of both Protestant and Catholic leaders revealed that such concerns were justified.[32] Any association of Perkins with the advocates of German race hygiene could easily destroy Anderson's ethnic survey. Perkins decided it was time to retreat from the front lines, regroup, and let others try to save the face of American eugenics. He reminded UVM president Bailey of his earlier request for a sabbatical for 1934–1935 prior to receiving Goddard's letter, and he resigned as president of the AES at their next board meeting. His colleagues urged him to stay on at least until the spring annual meeting. Perkins declined; "doctor's orders" was the only reason he gave.[33]

"It is well for us to be driven occasionally to take a cold-blooded, scientific account of . . . our program," Perkins had concluded in 1933, "compare it with the demands of the day, and then proceed to tear down, to rebuild, to add on until we have the best possible working plan for our enormously important enterprise."[34] Perkins's sabbatical furnished him with the opportunity to ponder his own role in such an endeavor and to leave Elin Anderson, as interim director of the Eugenics Survey, to work out the details. He did not attend the annual meeting of the Eugenics Research Association at Cold Spring Harbor, where Clarence Campbell, Perkins's former colleague and president of the Eugenics Research Association, stepped up his campaign for stricter race hygiene measures in America. In the fall of 1934, Perkins took his wife and daughters to Europe for a seven-month tour of England and the Continent, where he visited European museums and eugenics societies. Meanwhile, Huntington and Osborn finished revising the AES catechism, and Elin Anderson, her multicultural staff, and Eugenics Survey secretary Anna Rome Cohen, with Shirley Farr's renewal of financial support, conducted personal interviews of over four hundred Burlington citizens on their attitudes toward interracial relations.[35]

1935: Divergence

Perkins's sabbatical year proved to be a watershed in the history of eugenics. While he traveled abroad, eugenic sterilization of the handicapped was reviewed and debated in professional journals and state legislatures, and Hitler's race hygiene policies became the focus of scientific controversies over the value of eugenics research and its applications in public policy. Both skeptics and proponents of eugenics considered the implications of the Nazi regime's effort to apply eugenics to the goal of creating a "master race." Some intellectuals and politicians adopted Clarence Campbell's race hygiene position after a fashion, to suggest that the strongest national defense against a German master race was to amplify eugenics measures in their own countries. Others viewed the exploitation of eugenics to reassert German world dominance as an unwelcome intrusion and a perversion of an otherwise meaningful research program. The shift in the meaning of eugenics was brought into sharper relief with the publication of scientific commentaries on eugenic sterilization and racial biology in the mid-1930s.

In 1934 the American Neurological Association appointed a committee, chaired by Boston psychiatrist Dr. Abraham Myerson, to study the theory and practice of eugenic sterilization in the United States. The Myerson report, completed in 1935 and published in 1936, found no scientific justification for *eugenic* sterilization; the relative roles of heredity and environment in mental deficiency were too complex and poorly understood to expect sterilization to solve these problems. Myerson still advocated voluntary sterilization, with the consent of parent or guardian, of individuals having been diagnosed by medical experts with specific conditions: Huntington's chorea, "congenital feeblemindedness," schizophrenia, manic depression, and epilepsy.[36] Curiously, Perkins kept his thoughts on sterilization to himself amid this new surge of commentary on eugenic sterilization. He probably was gratified that the Vermont sterilization law reflected Myerson's recommendations of sterilization on a voluntary basis after expert medical diagnosis. He was probably relieved to have been unavailable for comment when Leon Whitney's *Case for Sterilization* (1934) was released and attacked as an illogical "collection of unconsidered opinions" that made "no serious contribution" to eugenics.[37]

Political developments in Europe also forced eugenicists to take a position on the issue of race. In 1935 several influential and widely publicized scientific critiques of eugenics race research were published in response to Nazi implementation of their race hygiene policies. Repeated citation of these works as evidence of the scientific defeat of eugenics has fostered a myth that knowledgeable biologists in the 1930s had abandoned any serious consideration of reproductive selection for the purpose of population improvement. The past decade of scholarship on eugenics, however, has revealed many of these scientific criticisms of mainline eugenics as integral to a reform effort by insiders, often on the political left, who were as dedicated as Perkins to eugenics. Like Perkins, many of the celebrated "critics of eugenics" had held racist or strongly hereditarian views in the decade prior to their apparent rebirth as antiracists or egalitarians in the 1930s.

Hermann J. Muller's *Out of the Night* and Julian Huxley and A. C. Haddon's *We Europeans: A Survey of "Racial: Problems*, both published in 1935, are the most frequently cited examples of the scientific defeat of eugenics as race hygiene. Because Muller and Huxley helped to draft the "Geneticists' Manifesto" in 1939 (the formal condemnation of Nazi eugenics and race science) and UNESCO's official rejection of biological explanations for racial inequality in the 1950s, their advocacy for eugenics is frequently overlooked.

American geneticist and Nobel laureate Hermann J. Muller, one of the most vocal critics of the American eugenics leadership, gave full expression to his concerns in *Out of the Night* (1935) in an attempt to liberate eugenics from its inherent race, sex, and class prejudices.[38] His opening remarks have been frequently cited as a rejection of eugenics in principle and its inherent connection with "race purification": "Eugenics, in the sense that most of us are accustomed to thinking of it, has become a hopelessly perverted movement . . . it does incalculable harm by lending false appearance to race and class prejudice, defenders of vested interests of Church and State, Fascists, Hitlerites, and reactionaries generally."[39] Yet Muller embraced the principal goals of eugenics and advocated reproductive selection for desirable human traits, as his full text reveals: "Thus it is high time for those who seek the real biological upbuilding of humanity to repudiate this perverted kind of 'Eugenics' and to devote themselves to furthering the economic, social, and intellectual changes which alone will afford the means of eventually undertaking a real biological upbuilding."

Muller firmly believed in the genetic basis of human nature and held that mankind's direction of its own evolution would ultimately rest on the precise diagnosis of genetic factors and their artificial selection through the application of reproduction technologies of the future. He predicted, for example, that "ectogenesis" (in vitro fertilization and gestation in artificial wombs) would free women from the burdens of pregnancy. He advocated sterilization for bearers of mental or physical handicaps, whose conditions had been proved to be genetic in origin. The confusion of hereditary and social factors in most eugenics research and policies, in Muller's opinion, had obscured the true path of eugenics. Absolute equality with respect to race, sex, and class must be achieved before an individual's true genetic potential could manifest itself. Muller, a member of both the National Academy of Science in the United States and the Academy of Sciences of the Soviet Union, advocated communism as a prerequisite for a sound eugenics program and turned eugenics into a political challenge: "It is easy to show that in a paltry century or two . . . [It will be possible] for the majority of the population to become of the innate quality of such men as Lenin, Newton, Leonardo, Pasteur, Beethoven, Omar Khayyam, Sun Yat Sen, Marx (I purposely mention men of different fields and races) or even possess their varied faculties combined.[40] Despite his undisputed expertise in genetics, Muller's glorification of the social experiment in the Soviet Union had little appeal for his colleagues in the United States. While attention was paid to his criticisms of "capitalist eugenics," his "Bolshevik Eugenics" engendered more derision than serious discussion.[41]

Julian Huxley, one of the celebrated architects of the "modern synthesis" (the reconciliation of population genetics with evolution theory), also has been miscast as an opponent of eugenics, or his support for eugenics is simply ignored. Like Muller, Huxley had neither abandoned the movement nor faulted its fundamental premise of genetic selection. He simply concluded that the eugenics mission had been perverted by the exploitation of biology for right-wing political agendas. In a complete reversal of his racist commentaries of the 1920s, he published *We Europeans*, a full-scale attack on "scientific racism," particularly Aryan race theory and claims of Nordic *biological* superiority.[42] At the same time he defended the eugenics "core." His often quoted preface launched the assault: "One of the greatest enemies of science is pseudoscience. In a scientific age, prejudice and passion seek to clothe themselves in a garb of scientific respectability; and when they cannot find support from true science, they invent a pseudoscience to justify themselves. . . . Nowhere is this lamentable state of affairs more pronounced than in regard to 'race.' A vast pseudoscience of 'racial biology' has been erected which serves to justify political ambitions, economic ends, social grudges, class prejudices."[43]

Like Muller, Huxley argued that the "immediate task of humanity is to set its economic, political, and social affairs in order," and then, with continued research into human heredity and evolution, to seek to use that knowledge for improving the genetic health of mankind.[44] *We Europeans* merged evolution theory, European history, and anthropological data to argue that European ethnic groups were not biologically distinct populations (races) but were political constructions used by those in power to exploit people whose language, customs, and religion differed from their own. In Huxley's analysis, any region of Europe represented tremendous genetic diversity as a result of migration and interbreeding throughout history. The alleged superiority of any nation, as measured by its advancement in language, knowledge, and innovation, owed its accomplishments to biological and cultural diversity rather than to "racial purity" and genetic isolation. The concept of race as a basis for eugenic selection, Huxley concluded, was meaningless. In the wake of the "lamentable confusion between the ideas of *race, culture,* and *nation,*" Huxley argued, "the term *race* as applied to human groups should be dropped from the vocabulary of science. . . . Until we have invented a method for distinguishing the effects of social environment from those of genetic constitution, we shall be wholly unable to say anything of the least scientific value on such vital topics as the possible genetic differences in intelligence, initiative, and aptitude which may distinguish different human groups."[45]

Muller's and Huxley's opinions received considerable attention in academic and scientific circles. Having specifically targeted Nazi race hygiene as the most extreme perversion, the opinions of race hygiene enthusiasts, like Harry Laughlin and Eugenics Research Association president Clarence Campbell, were falling into disrepute. In 1935 the AES joined the opposition to Nazi race hygiene with its publication of the revised catechism, *Tomorrow's Children: The Goal of Eugenics,* and the pamphlet version Perkins had suggested in 1933, *A Eugenics Program for the United States.* Fred Osborn, disenchanted with the pro-Nazi sentiments of his colleagues at Cold Spring Harbor, joined forces with Ellsworth Huntington, Perkins's successor, commandeered the final revision of the pamphlet, and financed its production and distribution. Huntington apologized to Perkins for Osborn's appropriation of their project in his absence and requested Perkins to review the final drafts of the new catechism and suggest changes prior to their issue. Both publications offered an interpretation of eugenics that satisfied many American scientists' reservations about the "old" eugenics.[46]

Tomorrow's Children retained the old catechism format, while emphasizing its importance as a replacement for Leon Whitney's *Eugenics Catechism* of 1926.[47] The controlled dialogue of the new catechism opened with the question "Why are children the most valuable thing in the world?" Describing children as bearers of the "human germ plasm . . . the most priceless of resources," Huntington made eugenics over into a program for child development. Eugenics, defined by Huntington as the alliance of sociology and biology, provided the means to develop human potential through an enlightened understanding of the interaction of heredity and environmental circumstances.[48] In order to create a more inclusive, global eugenics, Huntington dispensed with the rhetoric of race and celebrated instead the power of "unconscious eugenics" in diverse peoples: the Maoris of New Zealand, the Hakkas of South China, the Mozabites of the Sahara (a Muslim nonconformist sect), certain Irish communities, the New England Puritans, and the Jews. In defiance of German anti-Semitic policies, Huntington placed the Jews in the "same category as the Puritans":

> No racial group has a more distinguished roster of great leaders. No other stands anywhere near the Jews in the length of time during which it has continuously produced such leaders. . . . [T]he Jews have periodically been winnowed by persecution and migration. Or else they have been strengthened in their religious zeal by the addition of zealous persons and the falling away of those who were weak in the faith. Thus strength of character and tenacity of purpose have become Jewish traits, even though the Jews are greatly mixed in racial origin.[49]

The new catechism responded to the criticisms of Huxley and Muller without embracing the socialist politics. Huntington's global focus and respect for human diversity abroad also diverted attention from racism in America. Ironically, in a subsequent section on immigration, Huntington supported the 1924 immigration quotas, invoking the overpopulation argument (that the United States could not accommodate huge influxes of immigrants and assure their assimilation without compromising the quality of the environment) and substituting cultural for biological discrimination (that the United States should restrict immigration from "countries whose standards and ideals are dangerously low").[50]

Tomorrow's Children failed to transcend the inherent elitism in eugenics.

Huntington remained concerned over the differential fecundity of "high quality" and "poor quality" married couples. The latter, those who had produced too many juvenile delinquents, high school dropouts, and neglected and presumably unwanted children should be discouraged from having children. Impediments to procreation should be removed for "desirable" families, those who demonstrated "emotional stability, strong character, sympathy towards other people, intelligence, adaptability, originality, . . . and personal responsibility for the public welfare." All families, Huntington conceded, displayed considerable variability in all of these traits, and their members could be found at all socioeconomic levels. Yet those individuals or families lacking these qualities to such a degree that they are generally "recognized as a detriment to the community," Huntington argued, should be discouraged from having large families.[51]

Huntington's proposals to correct such dysgenic reproductive trends substituted an environmental management approach for a social engineering one. Economic incentives and improvements in living standards might encourage educated, successful, and "socially responsible" couples to have more children and at the same time discourage procreation among the poor and dependent classes. Over generations, he predicted, "high grade" families would eventually dominate the American population. While the choice to bear children belonged to the individuals involved, Huntington admitted, economic and social incentives could influence couples to make eugenic reproductive choices. Income, gift, and inheritance tax deductions for couples with larger numbers of children would enable parents with higher incomes and higher expectations for their children to have more children and support them through college. Initiatives to discourage "unwanted children" and "unplanned pregnancies" among the impoverished, dependent classes included health and vocational education and birth control services (including sterilization as an "option," which "outdated laws" in many states restricted).[52] In cities, slums should be replaced with healthy suburban housing, and all states should work to provide opportunities for full employment. Huntington embraced the country life movement agenda for rural improvement as a positive eugenics program, perhaps inspired by Perkins's synthesis of their respective goals. Together, these strategies promised higher standards of living and economic security for all those who "choose to work" and provided incentives for those at the bottom of the social scale to follow the trend of the middle class toward smaller families they could realistically support in a modern society.[53]

While Huntington's new eugenics emphasized social factors, he did not exclude genetics. Research and education in human genetics and population biology were still the most important tasks of a eugenics society in a democracy, Huntington reasoned, as only an informed citizenry would make more socially responsible reproductive choices. He recommended the integration of eugenics principles into units on heredity and reproduction in high school biology courses. In grammar schools biology could "be taught in such a way that eugenic principles are evident." Government leaders, physicians, clergymen, and human service professionals should be educated in sociology and human genetics, if only through lectures and literature for the general reader.[54] Such an educational mission would create a base of public interest and financial support for urgently needed scientific research in specific genetic diseases. Collaborative research in genetics, population biology, medicine, and sociology, Huntington predicted, would yield a scientific understanding of the causes of the apparent disparities in human potential and achievement.[55]

Huntington concluded *Tomorrow's Children* by presenting eugenics, the ability to direct the course of human evolution, as "one of the five most momentous discoveries." The first four—hunting tools, speech, fire, and writing (and hence all other forms of indirect communication)—had given human societies the means to create agriculture and industry, the foundations of "modern civilization." The application of social and biological research would be the next stage of progress in man's control over the conditions that produced suffering. War, starvation, poverty, infanticide, and deterioration in the quality of life, according to the new catechism, were the consequences of natural selection operating under conditions of overpopulation. Eugenics, with an emphasis on education, economic opportunity, and responsible family planning, could provide the means to transcend these forces and to ensure that tomorrow's children were born free of mental and physical handicaps into healthy, happy, and stimulating homes.[56]

Despite the obvious biases in Huntington's works, the new eugenics catechism must be understood in relation to events in 1935. While one can find similarities with Nazi eugenics programs, contemporaries felt the differences were more important. Eugenics in Germany stressed the subordination of the individual to the state and the creation of a master "Aryan" race. "Positive eugenics" measures in Germany—such as allowances for large families, encouragement of early marriage, and subsidies to struggling farmers—were conceived for the explicit purpose of producing a population of "pure Aryans" and were merged with "race hygiene" policies directed against German Jews. The Nuremberg Laws of September 1935 formalized the anti-Semitic component of Nazi race hygiene, which dispossessed Jewish people of their citizenship, their homes and property, their means of self-support, and ultimately their lives. The German emphasis on "blood," race purification, and their destiny as a master race invoked more derision than sympathy from American biologists and carried ominous forebodings for a generation who remembered the Germany of World War I.[57] The new American eugenics catechism, which reduced sterilization to a method of birth control, admitted ignorance on the complex causes of mental illness and mental deficiency, and eschewed racism, attracted more scientists and intellectual leaders back to the AES.

Reviews of *Tomorrow's Children* and *A Eugenics Program for the United States* praised the society's more positive and benevolent eugenics, which recognized the complex interrelations between child development, sociology, and heredity. The new philosophy was received as a welcome departure from the ravings of "madmen and fools" and was compared to Julian Huxley's scientifically sound interpretation of eugenics. Reviewers, at times critical of the emphasis on environment at the expense of heredity, nevertheless praised the "pioneering group of leaders" of the AES as having demonstrated "the beginnings of wisdom." Robert C. Cook, editor of the *Journal of Heredity*, predicted the new AES program "may well represent a turning point in eugenical thinking in the United States."[58] Between 1936 and the onset of World War II, the AES continued to refine its position on the means and ends of eugenics in a democracy. Frederick Osborn expanded the reformed vision in later publications by advocating equal opportunity, respect for individual freedom, and political democracy as necessary preconditions for a sound eugenics. He even joined forces with antiracist Franz Boas, the most outspoken critic of eugenics in America, to create an American committee to combat scientific racism. Osborn's leadership, wealth, and commitment sustained the scientific reputation of the AES until his retirement in 1970, when it became the Society for the Study of Social Biology.[59]

In 1935, Harry Perkins returned to the board of directors of the AES and the Population Association of America. He supported the revised catechism and continued as a more silent partner in the reform of American eugenics. In contrast, Harry Laughlin and Clarence Campbell at the Eugenics Research Association openly supported German policies of exclusion. At the World Population Congress in Berlin in September, Campbell saluted Hitler, praised Nazi race hygiene policies, and supported their premise that Jews were a biologically distinct and inferior race. In the wake of the resulting publicity, Perkins may have been relieved that he had declined Campbell's invitation to serve on the Eugenics Research Association board of directors in 1932.[60]

If Perkins traveled to Germany or Italy during his sabbatical, he chose not to discuss it. His European travels, according to his 1935 faculty file, included only England and France. Perkins never resumed his previous national visibility within the American eugenics movement. Instead, in the fall of 1935, he focused his efforts on raising funds for Elin Anderson's continued sociological research for the Eugenics Survey. Most notably, he sought a publisher for her ethnic study, *We Americans: A Study of Cleavage in an American City*, despite its criticism of the Protestant, Yankee culture that he personi-

fied and had cherished all his life. Perkins recognized that Anderson's answers to the "immigrant question" were an important contribution to the
reformation of American eugenics and, at the same time, a necessary demonstration of the Eugenics Survey of Vermont as a notable exception to the
more sinister elaborations of eugenics doctrine elsewhere.[61]

Because scholars received and reviewed *We Americans* as a study in social
anthropology rather than a contribution to the 1930s debates over eugenics
and because it presented such an extraordinary challenge to Perkins's own
eugenics commentaries, historical accounts of Vermont eugenics have persistently disregarded this work except for culling Anderson's files for racist
remarks to suggest strong associations of the Eugenics Survey with Nazi race
hygiene. Not only has this disregard led many to interpret the Eugenics Survey as a precedent for the Holocaust, but it has also repressed the actual historical trajectory of the Eugenics Survey's four-year investigation and resolution of the eugenic significance of "race." Attempts to explain the historical
forces that motivated Perkins's promotion of eugenics or the reason the University of Vermont in Burlington emerged as a center for eugenics, should
begin with Elin Anderson's *We Americans* instead of ignoring it. There is no
more definitive demonstration of the social and cultural forces that nurtured
Perkins's attitudes or a more courageous exposé of the sources of insecurity
that drove his eugenics research and education. His remarkable support for
her work attests to how clearly he understood the political vulnerability of his
organization in 1935 and the "tragic flaw" of his earlier teachings. (Fig. 4.2.)

We Americans: A Vermont Response to Eugenics Elsewhere

Anderson's ethnic study was originally intended to be published as the Eugenics Survey's sixth annual report. The scope of her investigations and their
political implications in 1935 called for a far more extensive analysis. Perkins
was anxious to get the study published and sent her manuscript to his colleague Ellsworth Huntington for his review while she completed the final
chapters. On the recommendation of Robert S. Lynd (and perhaps Huntington), Harvard University Press agreed to publish it as part of their new initiative to issue books that interpreted scholarly research to the "intelligent
reading public," not simply the usual "barren displays of erudition" emanat-
ing from academe. *We Americans: A Study of Cleavage in an American City*
(1937) offered a sociological perspective on the problem of ethnocentrism as
it manifested itself in rural America. Robert S. Lynd had suggested the title,
perhaps inspired by the parallel between Huxley's broad analysis of racial factors in *We Europeans* and Anderson's comprehensive demonstration of the
same phenomenon, in microcosm, operating within a New England town.[62]

4.2 Elin Lilja Anderson (1900–
1951). From *Rural Health and Social Policy*,
a testimonial in her memory published by her
friends and colleagues, Washington, D.C.,
11 June 1951. Courtesy Special Collections
Department, University of Vermont Library.

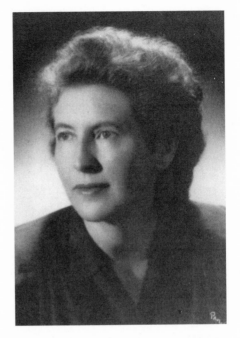

We Americans was a skillful blending of three levels of extensive research
into an articulate documentary of Burlington life in the style of the Lynds'
Middletown. Conventional sociological and demographic analysis provided
the infrastructure for Anderson's own observations, based on fieldwork inspired by her own experiences within the inner circle of Vermont's social
work network and the VCCL. Statistics and observations together would provide the background against which she laid the centerpiece of her study, the
interviews of a cross-section of the six largest ethnic groups in Burlington:
French Canadians, Irish, Jews, Germans, Italians, and "Old Americans." Anderson's initial purpose, according to Perkins in 1932, had been to examine
the eugenical significance of "racial factors" operating in Burlington. By 1935
the meaning of such a study had dramatically changed.

Anderson introduced her study as a response to the violent expressions of
fear and distrust that had erupted out of the economic insecurity of the Depression and the political instability emerging with communist agitation in
America. The lynching of Negroes by the Ku Klux Klan, protests of California
workers against the immigration of Asians, the terrorization of Jews, Catholics, and Communists by American organizations modeled on Nazism—all, in
Anderson's view, were symptoms of deeper antagonisms that had developed
naturally within a country founded on the idea of a common destiny among
diverse peoples. One expression of Americans' confusion over their identity,

Anderson suggested, was the enactment of such "patriotic laws" as compulsory saluting of the flag and prohibition of certain subjects in public schools.
Such reactionary measures, Anderson cautioned, contributed to "a dangerous narrowing of the definition of 'Americanism' which is at variance with the
very principles on which America was founded."[63] The search for scapegoats
to explain American insecurities and to "find in the alien the root of all evil,"
Anderson contended, "has led many to speak of that mythical figure the
'pure' American, a genetic concept even more anomalous than the 'pure'
Aryan." Within this paradox, between American promises of freedom and
opportunity and the social realities traditional American communities offer,
Anderson laid her ethnic study of Burlington.[64]

Anderson presented the city of Burlington as an ideal community in which
to examine these tensions. Its reputation, its history, and the image its leaders
had projected was that of a "Yankee town," the living tradition of American
ideals of freedom, individualism, and rural democracy. But in reality, as her
demographic study showed, the town had grown gradually, almost imper-
ceptibly, into an ethnically diverse city where Jews and Catholics comprised
66 percent of the population and the "pure Yankees" within the remaining
Protestant 34 percent made up "an extremely small part of the population."[65]
Because Burlington's ethnically diverse population had evolved gradually and
the ethnic makeup had not changed significantly in the past two generations,
Anderson assumed that the effects of immigrant assimilation were well established. Gradual population growth, accompanied by increased ethnic diversity, Anderson observed, had resulted in various groups assuming different
roles and identities. Despite the growing numbers of non-Yankees, foreign
immigration had never been great enough to threaten the power and privilege of the Old Americans, who, through their institutions, "set an indelible
stamp on the life of the community."[66]

Huxley and Muller had argued that the first task of eugenics was to create
an equitable society free of political, racial, and class prejudice in order that
individual genetic potential could be expressed. In *We Americans*, Anderson
analyzed the process by which social institutions, geographical boundaries,
and economic stratification reflected and reinforced the invisible boundaries
of racism, religious prejudice, and class consciousness that had evolved as
successive waves of European immigrants made their home in America. According to her central argument, cultural attitudes and values, reinforced by
historical legends and events, confer a sense of group belonging and identity,
which gives rise to ethnocentrism. When group identity and its defining values become established within social, civic, and religious institutions, cleavages among diverse groups deepen and create a climate of prejudice, fear,
and distrust, the chief obstacles to cooperation and unity. In Burlington this
process had prevented more recent immigrant groups from freely develop-

ing and expressing their own potential and the more established Vermonters, especially the Old Americans, from recognizing it.

By adopting Muller's and Huxley's politically liberal paradigm of eugenics as her basic premise, Anderson accomplished a dual task of dispensing with the eugenicists' classic obsession with "racial integrity" and postponing any further discussion of eugenics to some time in the future when Vermont had become the reality, not just the symbol, of American freedom and opportunity. Anderson jettisoned the race hygiene problem simply by definition. The proper term for the European nationals and those whose identity was derived from a cultural heritage beyond America was "ethnic group." For convenience, Anderson would refer to the Jews, like the Old Americans, as an ethnic group, recognizing their proper designation as a socioreligious group of diverse national and racial origins. Anderson accomplished the second goal by offering the new interpretation of eugenics as the rationale for her study, a tactic Perkins would have appreciated, having done it so many times himself. Acknowledging the Eugenics Survey as her sponsor, Anderson explained: "The eugenist is interested in the American problem of ethnic adjustment primarily in terms of the biological blending through intermarriage of the most desirable qualities of peoples. Yet because he finds that racial and religious prejudices frequently stand in the way of any ideal biological blending, his first task becomes the understanding and elimination of the environmental causes of such prejudice." But Anderson, the assistant director of the Eugenics Survey of Vermont and eugenics instructor at the state university, did not rule out eugenics: "Hence such a study as this, whatever sociological purpose it may serve, is an attempt at providing some groundwork upon which may be built a eugenic program of the future, based upon the full and uninhibited appreciation of the intelligence, special abilities, and social qualities of our diverse peoples."[67]

Affirmation of ethnic diversity as a potential source of community enrichment and creative solutions to common problems would provide the new cornerstone to build a eugenic Burlington. What had to be torn down were the dysgenic forces of racism, nativism, and religious hatred that had been constructed over time as Burlington had grown into a multicultural city. What was required, in Anderson's analysis, was for Vermonters, particularly the Old Americans, to reflect seriously on the extent to which they lived according to their celebrated tradition of tolerance and their professed ideals— "Freedom and Unity." After her introduction, however, Anderson never mentioned eugenics again nor placed her findings within a recognizably eugenic framework. Instead, she presented both a powerful indictment of the ethnocentrism that had colored all previous projects of the Eugenics Survey and a deconstruction of Burlington's mythical identity as a Yankee town. *We Americans* thus transformed the meaning of eugenics in Vermont by replacing the characteristic angst over the "alien in our midst" with a warning of the far more dangerous (and dysgenic) force of "the bigot in our midst."

This historic transformation was a product of Anderson's innovative approach to the immigrant question, her commitment to the philosophy of community cooperation, and, ironically, a logical extension of the precedents for eugenics research in Vermont that Perkins had set himself. It was Perkins, initially, who had broadened the scope of eugenics beyond the confines of biological explanation and brought local history and sociological analysis to bear on eugenic questions. Even in his 1928 plan to study French Canadian Vermonters, Perkins had buried eugenic concerns with birthrate and racial characteristics under the broader rubric of "citizenship" and an investigation of religious and cultural influences. Obviously, Anderson's answers to the "French Canadian question" were not the ones Arthur Estabrook would have offered had Carnegie sponsored his study of French Canadian Vermonters. But neither would Perkins have appreciated Estabrook's approach after 1933. Having embraced sociological explanations himself, he would have endorsed her consultation with Dartmouth professor Herman Feldman and her use of his *Racial Factors in American Industry* (1931) and other sociological studies of race to frame her study. Anderson addressed, implicitly at least, every aspect of Perkins's 1928 research plan that was relevant to the "new eugenics." In addition, she expanded her study of the "eugenical significance of race" to other immigrants: Jews, Germans, Irish, and Italians of Burlington.

Anderson added two important innovations of her own, which were extensions of her early work on rural migration and the VCCL philosophy of community development through self-study and cooperation. First, she studied the Old Americans in the same manner as all the other groups, as simply another ethnic group within the community rather than the American standard against which others were evaluated. Considering that they made up less than a third of the population, this was a logical strategy. She went one step further in leveling the playing field in her interviews. Through the opinion survey, she simply turned over the inquiry into the impact of racial factors on human development to all the people who were surveyed. The interviews enabled her to offer *We Americans* as the medium through which the attitudes and experiences of each ethnic group, in its relations with the others, could be shared. Their anxieties and struggles, their ideas and aspirations, and their diverse beliefs concerning intermingling and citizenship gave a human and personal quality to the otherwise distant statistical and factual information. Where prejudice existed, it frequently emerged in the interviews, and those expressing it condemned themselves. While her interviewees exposed the covert antagonisms reflected in the social and civic life of the city, many of them also confided their hopes for greater cooperation, acceptance, and respect, which many regretted finding only among their own kind. Giving all groups a voice in her study sent the message that their individual ideas mattered, thereby inaugurating the first serious conversation in Burlington that focused on the barriers of race, class, and religion with the intention of transcending them.

Anderson had launched her study the same year that Perkins had been promoting her fifth annual report as an exercise in "clearing up complications" concerning the "old Vermont stocks." From Anderson's perspective, one of the complications that needed clearing up was the attitudes of the old Vermont stocks toward immigrant peoples, particularly the French Canadians. Her survey would place that problem within the broader purpose of her study, which Anderson claimed was to consider "the extent to which rural America is united in the pursuit of common aims, and whether those aims are common enough so that such a community may face strongly the challenge of a changing world."[68]

Anderson's sociological and geographical data were consistent with most "melting pot" studies. The degree of upward mobility in wealth and status generally correlated with the longevity of particular families or ethnic groups in Burlington and the extent to which they asserted the traditions and values of their ancestral culture. Second- and third-generation immigrants tended to identify less with their foreign origins than their parents or grandparents had and intermingled more freely among other groups. Anderson's qualitative and anecdotal study of social, political, and cultural institutions brought the sociological data to life, and she offered her own editorial account of the experience of living in Burlington. She described Burlington's neighborhoods and political wards to illustrate the ethnic character of Burlington's social stratification. The elegant houses, spacious lawns, and arching elms of the exclusive Yankee neighborhoods stood in stark contrast to the neglected and depressing tenements near the mills and on the edges of town, occupied almost entirely by French Canadians. Colorful anecdotes enriched her observations of negotiated boundaries of race, class, and religion in commerce, the workplace, and politics. She explored the origins and propagation of religious cleavages in a comparison of parochial schools, where Catholic children learned history and citizenship in a religious context, with the more secular and patriotic traditions and curriculum in public schools. In her survey of worship, social life, and public life, Anderson revealed that the boundaries of race, class, and religion were complex, dynamic, somewhat permeable. She also found that the cleavages had become more accentuated during the post–World War I growth of institutions and social organizations, each serving different constituencies.

In *We Americans*, Harry Perkins's "fine old pioneer stocks" appeared a little less deserving and considerably less heroic than they had heretofore been portrayed. While Anderson had lived and worked as an "insider" for seven years within Burlington's Old American community, she did not share their parochial allegiances to Vermont's legendary past. She appeared to use Perkins's own words against him, as the Old Americans in *We Americans* were rendered, through the voices of her informants and her own conclusions, as an exclusive, "snobbish and ingrown" conservative group bounded by wealth, power, heredity, and race consciousness. They held all positions of trust and responsibility in city government, from the school board to the Department of Charity; they owned the banks and most of the manufacturing; and they resided in Burlington's most affluent and exclusive neighborhoods. Their cultivated historical identity with the founding fathers of the state had reinforced a "traditional feeling of the racial superiority of the Anglo-Saxon" and a "very deep conviction that the Protestant traditions of their forefathers are basically important to the development of free institutions in America." Their commitment to education and civic improvement were admirable in Anderson's estimation, but their persistent assertion of their own ideas and traditions as the best means to achieve those goals had exacerbated social and economic inequities and discouraged participation of non-Protestants in their "cooperative" ventures. It seemed to Anderson that the Old Americans were less concerned with social progress than with "nice living. . . . keeping their place and prerogatives; . . . and [putting] a check on too rapid an invasion from the lower ranks in society." No doubt it raised a few eyebrows among Anderson's sponsors to read how their own attitudes had contributed to the social problems that had occupied their attention for so many years. She softened the blow somewhat by framing her study as an analysis of a "process" rather than "criticism of any particular group of people or of a particular city" and by dedicating her book "[t]o Burlington in deep appreciation of what it is and of what it may become."[69]

Anderson found the French Canadian population to be the inverse of the Old Americans, not only in terms of wealth, education, and power but also in terms of their own understanding of their role within the community and their idea of good citizenship. The French Canadian community consisted of nearly ten thousand residents, including first- and second-generation immigrants and an even larger number of descendants from older French Canadian stocks. They had challenged the Old Americans demographically, but there their power ended. The poorest sections of town and the tenements were occupied almost exclusively by French Canadians, and French Canadians made up the bulk of charity cases and the working poor—mill hands, domestic servants, and menial and unskilled laborers. French Canadian representation and visibility diminished with each higher level of income and occupational status, becoming rare in the affluent neighborhoods, city administration, and the professions of law and medicine.

French Canadian social and cultural life took place almost exclusively within French Canadian Catholic parishes, schools, and charities, where the priest served as their guide in social, family, educational, and public life as well as in matters of the spirit. Interviews of the Irish and the Old Americans, in particular, revealed a prevailing opinion of the French Canadians as a complacent people, lacking strong leadership, ambition, and intellect yet quaint and charming in their simplicity. Yankees and Irish competed with one another for their allegiance, each claiming to be their advocates. The Irish more often expressed frustration with French Canadian complacency, while Old American prejudice took the form of paternalistic sympathy: "an attitude of an adult to a child, an appreciation of their warm, earthy simplicity, and a delight in the 'quaint' aspects of their behavior, as presented in the poems of Rowland Robinson." "But this attitude," Anderson noted, "is accompanied by a rejection of some of the very qualities that make them charming." While these sentiments surfaced in nearly all interviews of the Old Americans, they conformed precisely to Harry Perkins's own views, which he had confided to Anderson at the beginning of her ethnic study.[70]

French Canadians' interpretation of their civic contributions was somewhat different. French Canadian spokesmen countered that their apparent lack of achievement was really an expression of their belief that "the way of poverty is the way to heaven" and of their spiritual mission "to show materialistic America a way of life that is the way of Jesus."[71] In response to the interview question "What constitutes good American citizenship?" French Canadians gave the typical answers of the other groups—obey the laws, pay taxes, vote. But they were the only group that emphasized the view that "being peaceful with all other nationalities here is most important."[72] French Canadians, Anderson explained, did not consider themselves to be foreigners in Burlington. They viewed the Quebec border as an imaginary one. Their "peaceful penetration" into Vermont and its largest city on the shore of Lake Champlain simply followed the path of the French explorers and priests who discovered and began the first settlements. French Canadians' chief concern was maintaining what the Old Americans found most un-American in their culture—its language, religion, and customs. They passively and peacefully resisted Americanization as they asserted their claim on Burlington as a "French city" in the territory of their ancestors. In Anderson's words, "they put their faith in God and quietly produce the future population of the city."[73]

Anderson's study of Jewish Vermonters enabled her to draw attention to the problem of anti-Semitism in Burlington and use statistics and interview data to counter the stereotypes of Jews in anti-Semitic propaganda. The Jewish community in Burlington demonstrated a stronger commitment to social and civic improvement than either Protestants or Catholics and greater generosity, proportionately, in meeting the needs of the elderly, the sick, and the poor.[74] Their expressed desire to participate with Christians in the commercial, professional, and public life of Burlington stood in stark contrast to their experience of rejection and exclusion. Jewish teachers were not hired in Burlington public schools, the University of Vermont excluded Jews from its faculty and restricted Jewish students with "the Quota." Jews were actively denied admittance to many gentile neighborhoods and social clubs and were excluded from positions of leadership in government. Anderson admired the intelligence and self-reliance of the Jewish people and noted their rapid success in every aspect of city life where they had been granted the opportunity to participate. The Burlington Jews' experience of anti-Semitism, in its explicit and more hostile covert forms, invoked Anderson's sympathy. "With a long history of persecution and suffering behind them, they have sought to find a place of freedom for the oppressed. Perhaps the principles on which this country was based have meant no more to any group than to the Jews." She quoted one Jewish woman in her study: "The first thing I did when I came to America was to kiss the ground. This was a free land—my country. Here there would be no more pogroms."[75] In Anderson's view the discrimination against Jews was hypocritical for a community claiming to be the embodiment of true democracy and American ideals. But she found it to be dysgenic as well (although she did not use that term), in the community's failure to recognize, develop, and fully utilize the untapped reservoir of human talent in Burlington's Jewish population.

Aside from drawing attention to the racist remarks of some of her interviewees, Anderson did not explore the contributions of African Americans, Asian Americans, or Native Americans (Abenaki) to the cultural enrichment of the city. Her only reference to the presence of "Indians" was through the opinion of a banker of Old American stock who attributed the widely held perception of French Canadian inferiority to a belief that "they intermarried with Indians in the early days and so became irresponsible."[76] Anderson reported a general pattern among all groups in her survey: Burlingtonians preferred neighbors of their own ethnic identity. But it seemed to Anderson that the deepest antagonisms in the community were religious ones, within which all the others were submerged, and that religion was the issue Burlington citizens were most loath to confront. She found it paradoxical that some adult Sunday school classes wanted to promote better understanding of the "black and yellow races," while Protestants, Catholics, and Jews alike had made no attempt to engage in any interfaith discussions in which they would learn about one another's religious beliefs. In celebration of National Brotherhood Day, for example, each congregation prayed separately for peace and understanding among all peoples.[77]

In *We Americans*, the social problem group became the casualties of the competing interests and the resulting lack of cooperation among ethnic and religious groups. One would expect, Anderson contended, such differences to be put aside in attending to those in need: "The care of the poor, of the sick, of the delinquent, is a problem which should command the interest, if not the activity, of every member of the community. The extent to which these problems are shared is therefore an index of the community spirit."[78] The city of Burlington did not score especially well on this index.

French Canadians overwhelmingly dominated Burlington's dependent and delinquent population, just as Flint's study of poor relief had suggested and Anderson's own unpublished study of poor relief (1935) had validated. But Anderson dispensed with the old assumption that attributed French Canadian predominance on the charity rolls and in the reformatories to some innate inferiority. Anderson cited instead the deep, enduring prejudice against French Canadians and the failure of wealthy slum landlords to maintain even minimal standards for their French Canadian tenants as the causes of their sustained degradation. Because French Canadians had dominated the labor population, Anderson found, they were most vulnerable to unemployment in times of economic depression. That fact alone was sufficient to maintain their numbers among "temporary dependents" and render them more vulnerable to lifelong dependency. Anderson traced the vicious cycle of prejudice, loss of opportunities, and impoverishment that had pushed larger numbers of French Canadians into the social problem group.[79] Anderson found that the Old Americans, who dominated the boards of private charity organizations and the Burlington Charity Department, were loath to support those they felt were "undeserving," hesitant to grant relief and thus encourage dependency, and quick to attribute French Canadian poverty to some innate inferiority.[80] Catholic charities were generally far more generous than Protestant groups in raising funds for their brethren in need. Yet Protestant self-righteousness was not the only problem. Anderson lamented the habitual resistance on the part of Catholic leaders to cooperate in Protestant-initiated efforts to reduce juvenile delinquency. She cited priests' warnings to their parishioners against joining organizations founded by Protestants, such as the Boy Scouts, boys clubs, or the YMCA. Anderson criticized as negligent the Burlington Cathedral priest's response to the high rate of Catholic delinquency. Ascribing the high rate of delinquency among Catholic youth to the fact that "they were not good Catholics," she believed, served only to absolve the priest himself of any responsibility for the problem.[81]

Anderson drew attention to the Catholic distrust of Protestant social welfare agencies, yet she circumvented the role her own organization and its sister agencies had played in the Catholic retreat from cooperative ventures, by virtue of their search for "unwholesome" family groups, child rescue efforts, and promotion of sterilization. She complimented the "step forward" of the St. Vincent de Paul Society and the St. Anne's Society to consult the Red Cross and the city Charity Department for information on their own clients, but she regretted that Catholic participation in the social service clearinghouse had been entirely unilateral. She did not publicize her discovery that Catholic charity organizations were not permitted to offer information on any of the families they served to the State Social Service Exchange and were ordered by the bishop not to cooperate with the Children's Aid Society at all after some unspecified incident in the 1920s.[82] Anderson opted for neutrality in this covert war by redefining the social problem group as *victims* of religious separatism, of mutual misunderstanding and neglect by the all agencies that had claimed to be their advocates. The tradition of charity, in which each group "takes care of its own," simply wasn't working. What was required, Anderson concluded, was "a fresh approach in which charity shall be looked upon not as a more or less unwelcome Christian duty, but as a grave social responsibility."[83]

With the possible exception of Anderson's support of intermarriage as a eugenic measure to promote cultural fusion, eugenics themes, language, and topics are conspicuously absent from *We Americans*. Anderson did not cite eugenics literature nor discuss heredity, population improvement, or family planning. For this reason, one is likely to forget or dismiss as irrelevant Anderson's role in the Eugenics Survey. While the political controversy over eugenics in 1936 was certainly a factor, her own files suggest that her suppression of eugenic issues was more a consequence of local problems. She had discovered in her initial interviews how powerful a wedge eugenics had driven between Burlington's Protestant leadership and the Catholic majority of the population, as the battle lines between Catholics and Protestants over eugenic topics (sex and marriage) had been silently drawn in Burlington's schools, charity organizations, and hospitals. And the main objections to intermarriage, Anderson discovered, had been on religious grounds. Religious differences, many of her informants believed, sowed the seeds of marital discord, religious confusion and loss of faith in the children, and alienation of the family from both religious communities.[84]

To raise the specter of reproduction in relation to civic responsibility or child welfare risked turning private hostilities into open warfare over the meaning of marriage, family, and citizenship. Eugenics education, after all, was an expression of secular teaching of Protestant beliefs. Removing eugenics from the agenda of building a cooperative community offered the only prudent strategy to dissipate the religious dissension that eugenics initiatives had fueled and thus break the stalemate in the social progress of the city. The futuristic and egalitarian eugenics of Julian Huxley and Hermann Muller or the "new catechism" of *Tomorrow's Children* needed a period of gestation— and Burlington needed time to heal the wounds of the old eugenics and outgrow its ethnocentrism—before public discussion of topics of eugenic relevance would be productive. Anderson mapped out the cleavages and barriers that had become more strongly fortified during the eugenics era and, having imposed ethnocentrism as an explanation, tabled any further public discussion of eugenics.

Anderson's final chapter, "The Way Ahead," indicted the "ideals and forces" within America that had made a "virtue of conformity" and had rendered Americans oblivious to the value of biological and cultural diversity to human progress. Measurement of human worth, according to one's conformity to idealized "American" standards and upward mobility within Protestant institutions, had created a climate that fostered an ominous ethnocentrism. Ethnocentrism, the "enthusiasm" for and "appreciation" of our own culture with a corresponding "ignorance" and "depreciation" of others, Anderson believed, was the chief obstacle to a eugenic Burlington: "For this reason the potentialities of our diverse ethnic populations have remained largely unrealized. Differences which might have been contributory to a general community have been permitted to become bases for distinctions in themselves. . . . The failure to see through our religious and racial prejudices and preferences, by which individual worth might be more justly evaluated, attests to the short distance we have moved from primitive society and its characteristics."[85]

Anderson's "Way Ahead" contained the implicit yet unreserved rejection of the tragic flaw of *Rural Vermont*, namely, its assertion of Yankee Protestant traditions and heritage as the model for future community development, an error from which her program of the future offered redemption. Burlington's Old Americans, Anderson argued, by their "insistence on conserving, rather than developing" and their tenacious hold on the leadership of the city were largely to blame for the social disparities, lack of success, or resistance to community cooperation of newer immigrant groups. "The Old Americans," Anderson charged, "though they may be tired of some of the responsibilities which accompany the satisfaction of holding power, are yet loathe to yield their place, privilege, or prerogatives to the newer elements." The future of democracy, she predicted, would depend on the development of an "interdependent civilization." In her final analysis, "the task ahead of such communities as Burlington is not to worship their virtues as absolutes but to realistically adapt them to the complex demands of a changing world."[86]

By setting the old problem of maladjustment right back on the shoulders of Burlington's elite, Anderson gave them a new mission and the responsibility, as intellectual, political, and financial leaders in the city, to initiate it. The "way ahead" for Burlington required a recognition that the celebrated history of Yankee Vermont had cast a shadow of social injustice and represented the dangerously narrow concept of Americanism, which, Anderson warned, fueled discontent, the emotional tool used by demagogues to divide a people. *We Americans* sent the Old Americans—and Harry Perkins in particular—the message: Heal thyself, and become the leaders that this multicultural city deserves and that you claim is your birthright.

Anderson knew better than anyone the vulnerability of Perkins's position. She may have sensed that the best strategy to jolt him out of his own ethno- centrism was to trigger the same insecurities and patterns that motivated his projects in the first place—his thirst for leadership and respect, his avowed commitment to civic cooperation and progress, and his habit of adopting any new and politically fashionable program when the old had become a liability. After Anderson had turned Perkins's exclusive neighborhood, his clubs, his Protestant culture, and his revered university (the last stronghold of Protes- tant Yankee conservatism) into a powerful "agency of social control" that stul- tified human development, she threw him a lifeline with her "eugenic pro- gram of the future." Perkins knew she had done him a favor, for her way ahead was also a way out of any identification of the Eugenics Survey of Ver- mont with race hygiene advocates, Nazi sympathizers, or anti-Semites. By ac- knowledging Professor Henry F. Perkins's "patience and faith" throughout the four years of her study, she gave him his cue, and he proudly assumed his role as impresario of her new program.

We Americans received the 1937 John Anisfield Award, a national prize for books promoting interracial understanding, and the first printing sold out in a few months. Eduard C. Lindeman, Anderson's professor at the New York School of Social Work, wrote the preface; he commended her study as an important demonstration of American cultural pluralism and her insights as "more true and more precious than mere knowledge." While describing *We Americans* as "a 'slice' of regionalism," Lindeman found Anderson's analysis of Burlington to be a superb demonstration of "all that is complex in our diversified American culture." Understanding and appreciation of this di- versity, Lindeman contended, offered the best defense against a society gov- erned by bureaucratic controls and the coerced uniformity of "civilizations accustomed to authority and infused with a mythical conception of the state."[87] If Harry Perkins had to forfeit his pride in the "the fine old pioneer stocks" and abandon the mythology of Burlington as a Yankee Town for the promise of Lindeman's "happy diversity" in Burlington's future, it was a sacrifice he seemed willing to make when he promoted Anderson's study as the new voice of the Eugenics Survey. In retrospect, certainly, *We Americans* became Perk- ins's "most cogent reason for carrying on" instead of "dropping the whole works" as Goddard had advised in 1934.

Demagoguery, meanwhile, had become an appropriate description of eu- genics research and education at Cold Spring Harbor. Harry Laughlin's fa- vorable articles on Nazi eugenics were rewarded with an honorary degree of doctor of medicine from the University of Heidelberg in 1936. In 1937 the Carnegie Insititution's investigation of eugenics research at Cold Spring Har- bor concluded in censure of Laughlin's work and the suspension of funding for eugenics research and publication. Perkins had evidently joined some of his colleagues in the AES in distancing themselves from the Cold Spring Harbor group, and Anderson's ethnic study had provided him with the opportunity to conclude his own association with his old mentor Charles Davenport, who had encouraged his study of racial factors in Vermont in the first place. In 1935 the Eugenics Research Association, typically patronizing, queried Perkins on the "present status of eugenics education" in Vermont and the possibility of his constituting a committee to "support the plan of a state society for eugenics research and education." Perkins might have been amused at this suggestion. He returned the letter with his reply to Davenport himself a few months later, apologizing for the delay. "At the present time I am afraid I have little to offer," Perkins explained. The Eugenics Survey's four-year study on the "racial derivations of the people of Burlington" was in need of a publisher. Perkins wished that he could go over parts of the findings with Davenport for his insights, as the study had found "some exceedingly interesting food for thought in attitudes of Old Americans to each of the racial groups and on the part of each one towards the neighboring groups."[88]

Davenport never responded, but if he ever read *We Americans*, he would have understood the bitter irony in Perkins's final letter to him. While reviewers commended Anderson and the Eugenics Survey of Vermont for *We Americans* and professors across America assigned it to their students, the Carnegie Institution had forced Harry Laughlin into retirement and closed the Eugenics Record Office. The Eugenics Survey of Vermont had redeemed its reputation in its final act, while Davenport's organization had ended in disgrace.[89]

Response to *We Americans*: Perkins' Progress

At age sixty it is unlikely that Harry Perkins abandoned his views of the innate superiority of the Old Americans or the sense of entitlement to "nice living" and patriarchal privileges that accompanied this identity. Nevertheless, his public stand on civic matters and their eugenic implications suggests that Anderson substantially influenced his thinking. Perkins publicly supported Anderson's work and privately (and falsely) took credit for supervising her four-year study. *We Americans* became required reading in his eugenics course. He had persuaded his advisory committee in 1936 to authorize the sale of equipment from the Eugenics Survey office to help finance its publication, predicting, "You are going to be very proud of this book when you see it." Anderson returned to her native city after the survey closed in 1936 to become executive director of the Family Bureau of Winnipeg. Perkins, having failed to obtain funds for her sociological study of other Vermont towns, took over Anderson's eugenics course and taught her new methods and insights.[90]

The year following publication of *We Americans*, Perkins delivered the Founders' Day address at the University of Vermont. The topic of his speech, "Arnold and Allen: A Comparison and a Contrast" suggests his continuing fascination with Vermont's heroic past and with distinguished Vermonters as bearers of superior germplasm.[91] Yet the content of his speech carried a different message from what one might expect of a man who had said ten years before that "blood has told." Instead, Perkins compared the breeding and accomplishments of Benedict Arnold and Ira Allen to revise his public position on eugenics. While both heredity and environment were enormously important, he noted, human success or failure depended on personal motivation: "Personality is the resultant of *Heredity, Environment, and Reaction*. The ultimately important question to answer is: How does one *react* to Heredity and Environment?"[92]

Perkins portrayed Benedict Arnold as everything the "old eugenics" found desirable. Arnold possessed the innate intelligence and drive to develop his talents into a spectacular military career. He was the beneficiary, as well, of a superior education and family connections that rewarded him with a position of trust and responsibility in the Revolutionary War effort. Ira Allen, in contrast, had "an uncelebrated ancestry," less military training than Arnold, and a somewhat dubious moral reputation. Yet, Perkins pointed out, Allen had remained true to his vision of a free and independent Vermont and had established a state university at great personal sacrifice. It was Allen, in Perkins's analysis, who pioneered the enduring Vermont commitment to the education of future generations so that they might have a better chance in life. Benedict Arnold, despite his advantages of birth, talent, and opportunity, had chosen the path of "self-interest, vanity and greed," which, Perkins concluded, "were their own undoing."[93]

It would appear that Perkins had transformed eugenics into study in personal choice and responsibility rather than heredity or environment. His focus on self-sacrifice for future generations was timely, as Nazi aggression in Europe escalated and posed a far greater threat to "tomorrow's children" than mental incompetence or poverty. Perkins encouraged his audience "to be generous in our judgments and to hold ourselves above the wholesale condemnation of a man or an institution . . . upon all who have had their faults and have blindly made their grievous mistakes. Severe in our own shortcomings, let us be zealous in the search for the best in our fellow men, recognizing and emulating merit wherever it may be found, even in a traitor."[94] Arnold's merits—his resourcefulness, zeal, and determination—had helped him to defeat the British at Valcour Island and to seize Fort Ticonderoga. His subsequent treachery four years later, Perkins admitted, was a choice Arnold made as a "free agent" rather than a consequence of either heredity or environment.

Was Perkins's Founder's Day speech a cryptic confession of guilt and a plea for forgiveness for his own choices in the past? Had he consciously projected the errors of his early eugenics sermons onto Benedict Arnold and his own reformed views into the celebration of Ira Allen? Whether or not he was conscious of it, his 1938 speech was a parable for his own situation. Founder's Day, it should be remembered, served the purpose of honoring Ira Allen and other founding fathers of the university, but Perkins's use of eugenic themes to explore the question of treason was probably not a coincidence. As a director of the AES, Perkins was certainly aware of the censure of Harry Laughlin and Clarence Campbell for their open support of Nazi race hygiene, yet he may have appreciated their contributions to the twentieth-century intellectual revolution known as eugenics. His public confession that heredity does not create virtue implies his appreciation of the scientific and moral flaws of his earlier teachings on eugenics. Whether Perkins had taken the path of virtue or treachery he would let future generations decide. Having received a grant from the Historical Records Survey of the Works Progress Administration in 1936 to process and conserve the records of the Eugenics Survey and the VCCL, he had been immersed in a review and description of the enterprise for a published guide to the collection. In retrospect, the original purpose and projects of his Eugenics Survey had a different meaning in 1938 than they had had a decade earlier.

In 1939, Perkins advocated the replacement of the tenements in Burlington's North End with better-quality housing for low-income families, as Anderson had recommended in *We Americans* and the AES had been promoting in their new catechism.[95] Students in Perkins's eugenics course had constructed a pin map locating the residences of Burlington's inmates of the reform school at Vergennes. The concentration of pins in the location of the tenement complexes in Burlington's north end, Perkins noted, "has something to tell us and we will have to listen to its message whether we like it or not, even if it affects our pocketbooks to do so. If we refuse, our children will have to." Juvenile delinquency, they found, had emerged in neighborhoods with poor living conditions, "overcrowded, unsanitary excuses for homes, unhealthy, wretched places to bring up children, hard to preserve a vestige of privacy, decency, morals." The child of those slums, Perkins tactlessly predicted, would grow up to become "a charge on the town, a drunken loafer, or a criminal." Claiming still to be "an ardent disciple of heredity," Perkins admitted he could not ignore the environment. Evidently, he could not ignore Elin Anderson's criticisms either. For the first time, he publicly acknowledged the connection between the plight of the poor and his own life of affluence and opportunity: "Many adults of today were children in those below average dwellings when some of us were more privileged youngsters 25 or 30 years ago, housed graciously and healthfully." He admonished the propertied classes of Burlington for opposing the urban renewal plan because of its cost, suggesting that slum landlords were more concerned with profit and short-term prosperity. Shifting the blame for juvenile delinquency from the defective germplasm of their parents to the neglect of Burlington's property owners and civic leaders may have been his only contribution to Anderson's "new program of the future," for his new eugenics lesson retained the same rhetorical style and fascination with indicators of defectiveness as his first sermon on eugenics.

Vermont Eugenics Becomes "History"

In 1940, the completed *Guide to the Eugenics Survey of Vermont* archive was sent to Washington, D.C., for review and publication. Perkins supervised the description of the investigations and wrote its twenty-five-page historical introduction, "Resumé of an Eleven Years Study, 1925–1936." Perkins's retrospective emphasized the survey's progress—from its early family studies in the 1920s to an enlightened revision of its program as new facts "came to light"—and commended the noble goal of human betterment and the benevolent intentions of all those involved in the survey.[96] Banished from this historical summary were the "degenerate families," the Pirates and Gypsies and Doolittles, and the negative rhetoric that characterized the initial family studies, which Perkins titled the "First Investigation." Instead, he attributed its purpose, methods, and assumptions to Harriett Abbott's training at the Eugenics Record Office and her familiarity with particular families investigated through her work in the Children's Aid Society. Perkins cited the pedigree work on Huntington's chorea (the only trait in their pedigrees verified as genetic in origin) as illustrative of their family pedigree work. He admitted that the draft board results had motivated their early research but claimed that the survey had changed its focus when the National Committee of Mental Hygiene had disproved both Vermont's high defect rate and the "only suggestion ever made" (that of Charles Davenport) concerning race as a factor in the draft board rejections.

Perkins lauded the Eugenics Survey's role in the passage of an "enlightened" sterilization law based on medical advice and informed consent, as opposed to a "punishment for bad heredity." Recognizing that scientists no longer emphasized heredity as the cause of mental disabilities, Perkins defended sterilization on the grounds that "deficient and delinquent parents furnish the wrong environment for their children just as inevitably as they pass on contaminated germplasm. The fate of the children is the same." Perkins regretted that the public had frequently misunderstood the survey's role as purely a fact-finding enterprise, asserting instead that the responsibility for discouraging marriage and reproduction of the genetically or socially handicapped belonged to the communities in which the afflicted families lived and the families themselves. The survey was not "an authorized agency for carrying out its own recommendations . . . administration was plainly outside its territory." While Vermont's sterilization law was an important contribution of his organization, Perkins reiterated that it was only one of many reforms in mental health services and community improvement that interested the survey. The VCCL was the Eugenics Survey's most significant project, according to Perkins, and Elin Anderson's *We Americans* was its crowning achievement in the application of sociology to eugenics research in Vermont.[97]

Anyone who read Perkins's reconstruction of the history of the Eugenics Survey might have concluded that it was *his* enterprise that had cleared away the old, unsubstantiated beliefs in Vermont's "pockets of degeneracy," in French Canadian or other immigrant inferiority, and in the hereditary causes of pauperism, crime, and feeblemindedness. Throughout the Guide to the Collection, the reader is reminded of the Eugenics Survey policy to protect the privacy of persons and families studied and never to reveal their identity, lest others thoughtlessly or maliciously exploit their misfortunes. If others, in the past or future, betrayed the confidentiality of those studied by the survey, then *they* (not Perkins, his staff, or his advisory committee) would be responsible for any unpleasantness resulting from the public exposure of the family secrets he and his workers had so carefully collected and guarded.

While Perkins's historical account of the Eugenics Survey sat on a desk in Washington, D.C., Europe plunged into World War II. Hitler had overrun all of western Europe and was laying waste to London in the Battle of Britain. The Vermont Children's Aid Society responded to the crisis by becoming an advocate for child victims of war. The U.S. Children's Bureau had given them the provisional designation as an agency that could assist in finding foster homes for European refugee children, the casualties of Hitler's expansion of his race hygiene program to all of Europe. With this new endeavor the Vermont Children's Aid Society, too, began to construct an institutional history in which they posed as heroes in the epic struggle against the ignorance and devastation of the twentieth century. While Perkins had carefully documented the role of all those involved in eugenics work in Vermont, the Children's Aid Society simply airbrushed their participation in the Eugenics Survey out of their public history. A 1940 article in the *Vermonter*, "These Are Our Own: The Vermont Children's Society Comes of Age," inaugurated this erasure.

During the 1930s many of the services of the Vermont Children's Aid Society on behalf of children had been assumed by the Department of Public Welfare (DPW) through federal grants. After 1935 the society functioned primarily as an adoption and foster care service. During this transition it gradually shifted its programs from search and rescue of children from negligent or "vicious" parents to family support and counseling so that children could remain with their relatives or with their biological parents under proper supervision. Perhaps Anderson's discoveries of Catholic censure of the Children's Aid Society encouraged the society to begin publicizing their efforts to place Catholic children in Catholic foster homes or as near to their biological families as possible.[98]

"These Are Our Own," a testimonial by Harold and Vonda Bergman, retold the story of the twenty-one-year history of the Vermont Children's Aid Society and urged Vermonters to look with pride on the work of this organization. Through its leadership in the state, "valuable human resources have been conserved and developed, hundreds of children have been given an opportunity for a decent way of life, and Vermont has been made a better place to live."[99] It was the Vermont Children's Aid Society, readers were told, that had first responded to the devastation of the influenza epidemic in World War I, that had provided support for families during the Depression, and that had brought federal grants into the state for Child Welfare Services, Aid to the Blind, and Aid to Dependent Children. Throughout its history, the society had met with dedication a multitude of requests for assistance from "parents, teachers, ministers, and neighbors . . . [concerning] dependent, neglected children with health or behavioral difficulties, the problems of unmarried mothers and their defenseless babies and of distraught and distracted parents."

Absent from this epic was any reference to the society's earlier preoccupation with "feebleminded women of childbearing age," morons, or the "immoral and vicious" parents who brought up their children amid degradation and vice. Nor did this testimonial mention the society's efforts to solicit reports of child neglect. Instead, readers learned that the Children's Aid Society caseworkers had always been on hand to "prevent the break-up of a home" through "an ounce of prevention applied at the right time."[100] Harriett Abbott, who had died in 1939, was memorialized for conducting mental testing and family casework on children in the custody of the society. L. Josephine Webster, who had become director of child services in the New York state Department of Social Welfare in 1934, was honored for her "pioneering spirit" in child welfare work in Vermont. Establishing the State Social Servce Exchange (now called the Vermont Central Index) was only one example of her leadership and vision in the interest of helping families. Despite Vermont's progress in child services, the society's president, Asa Gifford, cautioned Vermonters that the added responsibility of assisting refugee children required an expansion, not a curtailment, of services to all children. The problem of unfit homes for children had not disappeared, as the photograph illustrating Gifford's remarks showed, but in 1940 the "guardians of young

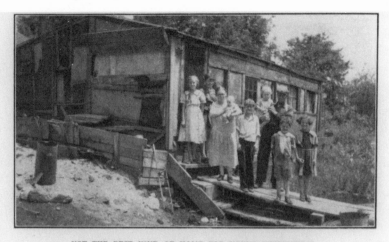

NOT THE BEST KIND OF HOME FOR YOUNG VERMONTERS
To "Guard Young Vermont" from the evil effects of living in homes such as this is one of the aims of the Vermont Children's Aid Society.

4.3 Juxtaposed with Dorothy Thompson's praise of the Children's Aid Society and Asa Gifford's warning, this family photograph captures the bitter irony of Vermont's eugenics history. From Henry Bergman and Vonda Bergman, "These Are Our Own: The Vermont Children's Aid Society Comes of Age," *The Vermonter: The State Magazine*, August 1940.

Vermont" sought remedies in the improvement of living conditions so that each child might achieve his or her potential. (See fig. 4.3.)

"These Are Our Own" concluded with a commendation of the Vermont Children's Aid Society from the famous antifascist journalist Dorothy Thompson: "Few Vermonters realize what wonderful work is being done by this society, which is a model for the whole nation. Its efficiency, incorruptibility, and brilliant management stands forth as a challenge to the totalitarians who claim they alone know how to take care of people. Vermont should be proud that here in this state, ready and waiting, is an organization worthy to look after the problem, not only of its own children, but also that of refugee children."[101] Thus began the celebration of Vermont family and child welfare programs as an antidote to tyrannical social engineering programs and the official forgetting of earlier collaboration with the Eugenics Survey.

The Vermont Children's Aid Society was evidently as eager as Perkins to relinquish its responsibility for the eugenic interventions in Vermont's once "notorious families." The omissions suggest a conscious repudiation of eugenics and an unstated recognition of its injustice. Suppression of the society's role in the family studies, unlike Perkins's historical reconstruction of it, was logical, perhaps motivated by the fact that the Children's Aid Society was still an active organization with a reputation to protect. Moreover, the society continued in the 1940s under the same leadership as it had had in the 1920s, with Asa Gifford as president and several of its charter members, including Eugenics Survey patron Shirley Farr, serving on its executive board. In 1941, Shirley Farr had taken up the cause of helping the immigrant refugees of the Third Reich and had provided a house in Brandon to shelter some of them.[102] Because access to the Eugenics Survey archives in the Fleming Museum was limited, members of the Children's Aid Society probably did not anticipate that their own documented supply of confidential family data to the Eugenics Survey would enter the public record.

Unlike the Children's Aid Society, the other arm of Vermont eugenics, the Department of Public Welfare, was staffed in 1940 by a new generation of social workers and welfare administrators with no direct connections to the Eugenics Survey. Instead of suppressing the history of past eugenics work in Vermont, DPW social workers exploited the Eugenics Survey records in the 1940s to promote their own agendas. With the infusion of federal money into Vermont, the state had established the desired welfare districts and traveling psychiatric clinics, and federal relief projects had put a number of destitute families back on their feet. In 1936 the DPW had assumed responsibility for the Vermont Central Index, the files of dependent families and delinquent or handicapped persons receiving public assistance or social services. These programs promised to achieve the VCCL vision of integrating "handicapped" persons into their communities with the support and supervision of qualified experts.[103] Yet, like the Mothers' Aid of 1918 and the surplus of neglected children collected by the Children's Aid Society and the Department of Charities and Probation in the 1920s, these programs soon had exhausted the available resources and overwhelmed social workers' capacity to realize their goals. The Eugenics Survey family case files and their exegesis in the DPW records provided evidence to explain the problems these social workers faced in rehabilitating many of the once "degenerate" families and their allegedly defective children. The new generation of child advocates inherited whatever damage eugenics had done or whatever problems Perkins and his colleagues had failed to alleviate. Despite Perkins's ten-year attempt to place the Eugenics Survey projects of 1925–1928 in historical context, the younger generation found the early family studies a suitable target for venting their own frustrations.

In 1940, Lillian Ainsworth, secretary of the DPW and chairman of the Committee on Legislation of the Vermont Conference of Social Welfare, conducted a survey of mental deficiency in the state. The long-awaited Society for Mental Hygiene in Vermont had been established earlier that year to develop mental health services in the state. Ainsworth began her investigation with the retrieval of the National Committee on Mental Hygiene

(NCMH) study of 1927 from the Eugenics Survey files. Perkins, she discovered, had been negligent in promoting the NCMH findings. Ainsworth reprinted the entire NCMH summary in her report, "Vermont's Feeble-Minded Problem," to document the unrecognized and long overdue need for a state program of control of the feebleminded. She criticized Perkins for failing to publicize the extent of Vermont's feeblemindedness problem more aggressively. Now that the state was hoping to discharge inmates of state institutions and many of those released had failed to make the expected adjustment to society, it appeared that the state had insufficient resources to supervise them within their home communities. While Vermont had fallen behind in their obligations to the feebleminded, Ainsworth argued, the NCMH study had become "nothing more than a museum piece in the Fleming Museum." She proposed that Vermont establish a program based on the South Dakota model, where a central state authority required teachers to report any evidence of mental deficiency or personality disorders and prescribed corrective measures ranging from special education to eugenic sterilization. In addition to expanding special education and fostering positive attitudes in communities toward the "underprivileged," Ainsworth recommended mandatory mental testing of public school pupils at registration and that "more serious attention be given to the problem of eugenics in this state." In response to her report, the General Assembly of 1941 created the state Board of Control of Mentally Defective Persons. Commissioner of Public Welfare Timothy Dale, who had authorized Ainsworth's study, chaired its advisory board, and Ainsworth became the secretary. Its first project, like that of the Eugenics Survey, was to "take a census of the defectives in the state."[104]

Social workers in Child Welfare Services and Aid to Dependent Children were also experiencing difficulties in turning dependent families into "self-supporting social units" and integrating "graduates" from the reform school in Vergennes and the Brandon Training School into community life. The Eugenics Survey had been a large part of the problem, they concluded in a fifty-five-page report, "What Mental Deficiency Means to the State of Vermont."[105] Their new survey of the old problems found the studies of "degenerate families" and interventions by the DPW from 1928 to 1942 to have been costly, ineffective, and inhumane. The public trust in the benevolence of social workers had been destroyed in some cases, and Perkins's negative publicity on the sources of Vermont "degeneracy" in the early annual reports had complicated the new agenda to secure community cooperation and acceptance of the previously condemned families.

"What Mental Deficiency Means to the State of Vermont" described the fate of one of the Eugenics Survey's "expensive luxuries," the "Doless" family (renamed the "Goodspeeds") to argue that "human problems require human solutions" and to indict the past practices of breaking up families and sterilizing problem children. In 1928 the truant and health officer of Pondville, Vermont, had requested the DPW to investigate the Doless family. A neighbor had complained that the younger children had been stealing from her, and their teacher had reported truancy, behavior difficulties, and child battering. The oldest daughter, seventeen-year-old Helena, had assumed the care of her six younger siblings because of her mother's poor health. The state social worker assigned to the case had arrived in Pondville to discover that the thirteen-year-old and ten-year-old had been sent to reform school for stealing, which Helena had encouraged. Helena's insolent response to the admonitions of the truant officer and social worker for corrupting her younger siblings had not helped the Dolesses' case. But their fate was sealed when Helena, in an act of adolescent defiance, proceeded to loot the complaining neighbor's house immediately after the visit. "When a family like the Doless family, that nobody wants, that is a nuisance in school, that is always an offense to the eye and the mores of the community, has a child that steals, something happens," one social worker complained.

After Helena's outburst she and the remaining Doless children had been sent to the Vermont Industrial School and the Brandon School for the Feebleminded. Three of the four oldest children, including Helena, were subsequently sterilized prior to discharge, and the three youngest at Brandon, "high grade morons," were soon to graduate with high marks and excellent character. Meanwhile, Helena had married. With the assistance of the government-funded Farm Settlement Program, she and her husband became productive and dependable citizens. Acquaintances remarked that "it was a pity she never had a family." The parents of these children had also been transformed into self-sufficient farmers through the Farm Settlement Program. Sad and bewildered that their children had been taken away by the state, the elder Dolesses made beloved pets of their farm animals, the surrogates for their lost children. Had the community and authorities offered a helping hand, this report concluded, instead of eight years of incarceration, seven years of parole, and dozens of evaluations by doctors, social workers, and public officials, the state might have saved money and spared this family's suffering.[106]

The goal of welfare work in the future, one social worker argued, should be to "remove causes wherever possible to improve our citizenry." In a lengthy critique of Goddard's theory of feeblemindedness and Perkins's first annual report, she urged the creation of a central state authority to diagnose mental deficiency, staffed with competent psychiatrists and more enlightened family caseworkers to avoid abuses of families like the Dolesses. Mental illness was a complex condition that had been casually misdiagnosed by eugenicists. Yet her main criticism of the eugenics-inspired welfare work was its expense and failure to achieve results. Vermont had produced only a few more "Goodspeeds," while many more "very prolific" families unable to support themselves were still a growing problem. Vermont required mental health programs to provide long-term solutions "that will preserve our dearly beloved Vermont for our men who go every generation or two to fight for it as something more than lovely scenes and natural delights, but as a place that is good to live in, a state of pleasant communities, the kind one wants to bring up children in and stay there all the days of their life." She invoked the wartime slogan "Save the Scrap—We Need It to Win the War" in reference to the money wasted on ineffective interventions, but the tenor of her report suggests she meant to apply it to Vermont's "human resources" as well.[107]

"What Mental Deficiency Means to the State of Vermont" documented three developments in eugenics history. First, the early eugenics work had in fact altered the relationships between welfare authorities and the families they served and created a climate of prejudice, which in turn invited interventions against particular families and ultimately justified "voluntary" sterilization of young persons on release from state institutions. Second, despite these social workers' denunciation of policies based on obsolete theories, they retained the core eugenic belief in reproductive intervention and family rehabilitation to "raise a better crop of children." At the same time, their revision of social work conformed precisely to the AES's latest revision of eugenics, published in *American Eugenics Today* (1939), which Perkins himself had co-authored. Finally, just as Perkins and his associates had done fifteen years earlier, the new generation of social workers exploited the ignorance and failures of their predecessors while embracing at the same time the latest research in eugenics, social psychology, and medicine to expand their own programs and enlarge their own influence over education, child development, and family life in the state. Their predecessors, for example, had not understood that Helena Doless's behavior was simply an adolescent phase, not a permanent condition. The Dolesses, in the 1940s diagnosis, were not congenitally feebleminded but suffered from "infantilism," a developmental disability of many families of the "submarginal" and isolated mountain culture. Because they married young and had too many children, they had become incompetent, immature adults due to lack of modern education and repeated assaults on their self-esteem by the communities that had rejected them. Eugenicists who had once attributed the Dolesses' circumstances to defective genes had ignored their history and the culture of rural isolation that explained their disabilities. Birth control clinics sponsored by Planned Parenthood, family counseling services, and public education concerning community responsibility to these unfortunates provided more progressive and humane alternatives for managing such families. Sterilization and segregation should be the last resort. Yet "What Mental Deficiency Means to the State of Vermont" still acknowledged that, for some families they served, such measures provided "the only solution."[108]

While Vermont social workers deliberated over the most humane and cost-effective means to managing handicapped Vermonters, the Third Reich had killed hundreds of thousands of handicapped children and adults, and the genocide of Jews, Gypsies, Soviet war prisoners, and "asocials" was reaching its climax. Whether Vermonters learned of the nature and extent of Hitler's final solution until after the war is unknown. They certainly saw no similarity between Nazi solutions and Vermont's revised approach to eugenics. In 1946, Frederick Thorne, state psychiatrist and superintendent of the Brandon Training School, attributed the genocide to the failure of a society to provide a compassionate and scientifically enlightened means to prevent the reproduction of "hereditary defectives." Vermont must face up to its responsibilities to the underprivileged, he warned: "There are others who would exterminate the unfit or support them on minima levels of existence oblivious to the inevitable human degradation which results from allowing any underprivileged group to grow like a cancer threatening the health and welfare of the whole society. The only alternative to the moral collapse which inevitably overwhelmed Europe following Fascistic methods of handling these problems is the development in America of truly enlightened methods."[109] Thorne and other mental health officials understood sterilization under Vermont law to be one enlightened option for some retarded persons, including the twenty who had been sterilized in his own facility over the previous two years. But Thorne noted that Vermont needed larger facilities at Brandon, another colony for feebleminded girls, and more psychiatric clinics in the state. "We in Vermont," Thorne cautioned, "must not fall behind in facing our responsibilities to the large mentally defective group while, at the same time, protecting society against the vicious circle of poverty, degeneracy, disease, and delinquency, which this group becomes involved in unless properly supervised."[110] It would appear that the best defense against fascist eugenics in 1946 was to expand the American version of it.

In 1945, University of Vermont president John Millis invoked the retirement rule, and Harry Perkins, along with all other faculty over the age of sixty-five, was forced to retire. Most of the affected senior faculty were embittered by this particular measure to get the university out of debt, and Perkins was no exception. He was honored, as his father had been, with a special ceremony at Ira Allen Chapel to celebrate his achievements. Henry Pratt Fairchild, Perkins's close friend and comrade in the liberal reform of American eugenics, gave the keynote address. Fairchild had continued on the executive boards of diverse organizations that embraced the new eugenics, many of which had grown out of the mergers he and Perkins had negotiated in the early 1930s. Fairchild's speech, "Population and Peace," outlined the new directions for the future: education in birth control, reproductive responsibility, and the problem of world overpopulation.[111]

Perkins passed the baton of eugenics education to his friend and re-spected colleague, Professor Paul A. Moody, who would teach the new eu-genics to the postwar generation. Moody, like Professor Fairchild and Dr. Thorne, presented American eugenics as the antidote to war and human mis-ery. In 1945 he had addressed the university during World Brotherhood Week. In his lecture, "Frontiers of Knowledge in Biology," Moody noted that mankind progressively had assumed the responsibility for his own evolution. World peace and the survival of the human race would require the "selec-tion" in favor of cooperative instincts rather than aggressive ones. In future centuries, man would "look back with repugnance upon the bloody dark ages of the Twentieth Century," Moody predicted, and live out Christ's prophecy that the meek would inherit the earth. As a member of the American Society of Human Genetics, an organization started by Hermann Muller in 1947 to place research in human heredity (and eugenics) on a solid scientific founda-tion, Moody embraced the effort to create a science of human heredity free of race and class prejudice. As a friend and colleague of Perkins since 1929, Moody understood most clearly the evolution of Perkins's eugenics philos-ophy and its connection with his own teaching of human genetics and evo-lution. He wrote Perkins's eulogy in 1956 and dedicated his textbook, *Genet-ics of Man* (1969) "[t]o the memory of my friend and predecessor, Henry Farnham Perkins, Ph.D., Founder and Director of the Eugenics Survey of Vermont."[112]

The closing of the Eugenics Survey in 1936 , followed by Perkins's retire-ment in 1945, brought an end to the official alliance of biology education, professional social work, and mental health programs in Vermont that eugen-ics had forged. Each institution involved in the Eugenics Survey indepen-dently retreated from the scientific errors of the family pedigree studies and absolved itself of the injustices that ensued, while the documentation of their activities lay safely buried in their confidential archives. Each institution had drawn the same conclusions regarding the old eugenics and adopted a phi-losophy consistent with the new eugenics that Perkins had helped to create. Unlike his associates Truman Allen, Guy W. Bailey, Harriett Abbott, and Elin Anderson, Perkins lived long enough to see his life work become "history." In 1952 a new curator of the Fleming Museum began to disassemble and de-accession the American collection that Perkins had created over fifteen years. Some artifacts were stored; most were sold, distributed to any department who wanted them, or simply discarded. The Eugenics Survey and VCCL archive was part of the museum overhaul. The books of the Eugencs Survey library disappeared into the UVM library collection, where most remain in a storage annex. The bulk of the archive might have ended up in the city dump, had it not been rescued by Director of State Public Records Olney Hill, who sensed its historical value and found a storage place for it in his division.

In 1955 the editor of *Vermont History* asked Harry Perkins to tell the story of the VCCL, whose product, *Rural Vermont*, had a "lasting effect on the destiny of the State, [and] . . . belongs in the history of Vermont.[113] Perkins recounted the origin of the Eugenics Survey, its abandonment of the studies of degenerate families, and its evolution into the VCCL when he and his associates recognized that the real problem of rural decline lay in substandard living conditions rather than bad heredity. Perkins noted the importance of cooperation among diverse groups within the state and with the national organizations that provided endowments. While giving himself credit for the original idea, he praised the achievements of others, particularly the leadership of VCCL director Henry C. Taylor, whose expertise and insights guaranteed its success. Some aspects of the survey had been controversial, Perkins admitted. Yet Vermonters' willingness to confront problems in state services had led to improvements. The example he cited was the report of the Committee on Medical Care, which had exposed inadequacies in hospital and health services in some parts of the state. Perhaps this last commendation was a silent memorial to Elin Anderson, who had died of cancer in 1951 at the height of her career, developing community health services in rural America.[114]

Perkins noted that the VCCL findings needed review, and perhaps a new comprehensive study was in order, an idea that had been suggested in 1952 and abandoned as impractical. Yet he felt that the ideas of the original survey were still very much alive, as "*Rural Vermont* [had] become the source for much progressive thinking in the state." That two hundred Vermonters had collaborated to study, define, and discuss the issues of rural life and "the common problems of the state as a whole" was the most important aspect of the enterprise.[115] In 1955, form and process evidently were far more important than the specific content of *Rural Vermont*.

It is not surprising that Perkins was silent on the eugenic agenda of the comprehensive rural survey. The entire world was silent on the topic of eugenics in the early 1950s. Americans were perhaps too preoccupied with defining themselves in opposition to totalitarianism and celebrating their freedom through honoring the sacrifices of those who had fought for it. They preferred the Norman Rockwell visions of happy, wholesome, American families and peaceful communities to reflections on social injustice. Tragically, there were war veterans who would not share in the sentimental scenarios depicted in Norman Rockwell's Four Freedoms and his nostalgic celebrations of small-town Vermont life. While they had been found sufficiently fit to fight in 1941 for the freedom and security of "tomorrow's children," either they or their wives had been deemed unfit to conceive or raise them, according to the scientific and medical consensus of the interwar years. Childless, they would watch the baby boom generation enjoy unprecedented indulgence and prosperity. Most of them kept the secret as well, too humiliated perhaps to divulge the reason that they had no children.[116]

Henry Perkins died in 1956 at the dawn of a new age. The discovery of the structure and action of DNA had just been published. In 1956 the first karyotypes of human chromosomes had been made, enabling researchers to discover abnormalities in chromosome numbers and structure. From these discoveries scientists would develop the means to demonstrate and diagnose the genetic source of many human diseases and traits with more certainty and authority than Perkins could have imagined. The eugenic consciousness that Perkins predicted in 1933 and instilled through twenty-five years of public and university education would reawaken, as would the old questions on the social applications of human genetics research. But after 1970 interdisciplinary collaborations on these issues would be called by some other name than eugenics.

Appendix A: The People and Projects of the Eugenics Survey of Vermont

Henry F. Perkins, Director (and Chairman, Advisory Committee)

Staff

Harriett E. Abbott (1925–1927): Family studies, pedigrees

Francis E. Conklin (1927–1928): Family studies, "Better Branches"

Martha M. Wadman (1928–1929): Key Family Study, Town Study; Rutland Reformatory Study; Brandon Waiting List

Elin L. Anderson (1929–1936): Assistant Director, 1931–1936; Instructor of Eugenics, 1932–1936; Migration Study, *Fifth Annual Report*, 1931; Ethnic study of Burlington, *We Americans*, 1937

Marjorie Choate (1930–1931): Migration study

Anna Rome (Cohen) (1926–1936): Secretary; Field Assistant, Town, Migration, and Ethnic studies

Advisory Committee°

Guy W. Bailey, President, University of Vermont
  Treasurer, Vermont Children's Aid Society

Asa Gifford, UVM Sociology Professor
  President, Vermont Children's Aid Society
  Chairman, Vermont Conference of Social Welfare Legislative Committee

K. R. B. Flint, Norwich University
  Professor of Political Science
  Director, Bureau of Municipal Affairs
  Author, *Poor Relief in Vermont*, 1916

Dr. Truman A. Allen, Superintendent, Vermont State School for the Feebleminded

Dr. E. A. Stanley, Superintendent, Vermont State Hospital for the Insane

Charles W. Wilson, Superintendent, Vermont Industrial School

Lena C. Ross, Superintendent, Riverside Reformatory for Women

R. H. Walker, Superintendent, Vermont State Prison

Dr. Horace G. Ripley, Superintendent, Brattleboro Retreat

°Served during 1925–1932, not all members listed attended meetings

Dr. C. F. Dalton, Secretary, Vermont State Board of Health
William H. Dyer, Commissioner, Vermont Department of Public Welfare
Clarence H. Dempsey, Commissioner, Vermont Department of Education
Shirley Farr, Incorporator and member of Executive Board,°°
    Vermont Children's Aid Society
    Eugenics Survey benefactor, 1926–1936
Josephine Webster,°° General Secretary, Children's Aid Society

°°Served 1928–1932

Appendix B: An Abbreviated Family History, 1925

One of the first family pedigree studies, this one was prepared by Charles Wilson and Lena Hamilton at the Vermont Industrial School in 1925 (the text accompanying the chart is reproduced on pp. 182–183). By September 1926, Harriett Abbott had traced the family back six generations and expanded the pedigree to include 297 relatives. By 1927 she had estimated the expense for charity and incarceration to be $59,608 for Vermont and neighboring states. Further genealogical study connected this family with the "Rectors," one of Francis Conklin's "Better Branches" featured in the Eugenics Survey's third annual report (1929). Special Pedigrees Complete, ESV papers. Courtesy of Vermont Public Records Division, Middlesex, Vermont.

PEDIGREE CHART

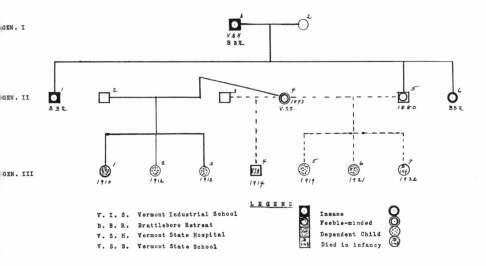

THE HEREDITY

(Gen. II #5) is (in 1926) 46 years old. He is illiterate, feebleminded, a sex offender and a wanderer. His father (Gen. I #1), his brother (Gen. II, #1) and his sister (Gen. II #6) were insane and were in institutions for the insane in Vermont for many years.

(Gen. II #4) is (in 1926) only 33 years of age. She is feebleminded and a serious sex offender. She comes of a very prolific family in which a low grade of intelligence, sex offenses and general shiftlessness are the predominating characteristics.

THE HISTORY
of
(Gen. II #5) and (Gen. II #4)

(Gen. II #4) married when she was fourteen years old and was deserted a few years later. She then lived with many different men. We have records of seven children. There were probably more. When she was 26 and was the mother of three living children, she and (Gen. II #3) were arrested for adultery in Massachusetts. She and her paramour were in prison for about a year and while there she gave birth to (Gen. III #4). Ever since her imprisonment the State of Massachusetts has taken charge of her children (Gen. III #1, #2 and #3).

Since her release from prison she has had at least three children by (Gen. II #5) with whom she lived in conditions which were of the worst physically and morally.

In 1922 she was committed to V. S. S.

(Gen. III #4) became delinquent and at the age of eight was committed to V. I. S. He is of low mentality.

(Gen. III #5) and (Gen. III #6) are dependent on a Vermont town and are wards of the Vermont Children's Aid Society.

THE FUTURE

(Gen. II #4) is in the V. S. S. colony. While thus protected she becomes more and more efficient and costs the state less and less.

(Gen. II #5) is at large and is living with another woman and is probably still passing on defective germ plasm.

(Gen. III #1, #2 and #3) are only 16, 14 and 13 years of age respectively and will continue to cost the State of Massachusetts $260 a year for some years to come.

(Gen. III #4) is only 12 and will continue to cost the State of Vermont over $500 a year for many years. (Gen III #5) and (Gen. III #6) are only 7 and 5 years of age respectively (in 1926). Although mental tests show them to be of normal intelligence, they cannot (because of their heredity) be placed for adoption and will for many years to come continue to cost their town $200 or more each year.

THE EXPENSE
of
(Gen. II #4) and (Gen. II #3)
(and the descendants of)
(Gen. II #4)
1914–1926

	VERMONT	MASS.	TOTAL
Gen. II #4	$1553.94	$ 245.14	$ 1799.08
Gen. II #3		40.60	40.60
Gen.III #1,#2,#3		8821.11	8821.11
Gen.III #4	2343.58	183.00	2526.58
Gen.III #5	567.00		567.00
Gen.III #6	988.75		988.75
	$5453.27	$9289.85	$14743.12

Appendix C:
Vermont's Sterilization Law, 1931

No. 174—An Act for Human Betterment by Voluntary Sterilization

It is hereby enacted by the General Assembly of the State of Vermont:

Section 1. *Construction*. Henceforth it shall be the policy of the state to prevent procreation of idiots, imbeciles, feeble-minded or insane persons, when the public welfare, and the welfare of idiots, imbeciles, feeble-minded or insane persons likely to procreate, can be improved by voluntary sterilization as herein provided.

Section 2. *Examination and certificate; operation; report*. When two physicians and surgeons legally qualified to practice in the state, examine a person resident of the state, and decide: (1) that such person is an idiot, imbecile, feeble-minded or insane person likely to procreate idiots, imbeciles, feeble-minded or insane persons if not sexually sterilized; (2) that the health and physical condition of such person will not be injured by the operation of a vasectomy, if a male, or a salpingectomy, if a female; (3) that the welfare of such person and the public welfare will be improved if such person is sterilized as aforesaid; and (4) whether such person is or is not of sufficient intelligence to understand that he or she cannot beget children after such an operation is performed; and they make and sign duplicate certificates setting forth those facts and make oath thereto before a justice of the peace or notary public, then it shall be lawful for any other physician or surgeon, legally qualified to practice in the state, when presented with such certificate, to perform such operation provided: (1) he decides that the public welfare will be improved by such operation; (2) such person has requested in writing, on such certificates, that said operation be performed, if the certificates show that such person is of sufficient intelligence to understand that he or she cannot beget children after such an operation is performed; or (3) the natural or legal guardian of such person has requested in writing on such certificates that such operation be performed, if certificates show that such person is not of sufficient intelligence to understand that he or she cannot beget children after such an operation is performed; and (4) such person voluntarily submits to such operation. The physician and surgeon, after performing such operation, shall endorse on each of the duplicate certificates, when and where he performed such operation, keep one of the certificates, and mail the other, postage prepaid, addressed to the commissioner of public welfare, at Montpelier, Vermont, to be kept in his office.

Section 3. *Inmates of state institutions; fee.* If such person is being supported by the state in any institution in the state, the commissioner of public welfare is authorized to contract with two competent physicians and surgeons, not in the employment of the state, to examine such idiots, imbeciles, feeble-minded or insane persons as he has reason to believe should be sterilized, at the price not exceeding three dollars for each physician and surgeon, and if they make the certificates aforesaid, then the said commissioner is authorized to contract with a competent physician or surgeon, not in the employment of the state, to do such operation at a price not exceeding twenty dollars for males and thirty dollars for females and to contract with the hospital for such care and nursing of such person as necessary, at reasonable prices, and such expenses shall be paid by the state and charged against the appropriation for the support of the institution supporting such person.

Approved March 31, 1931.

(*Laws of Vermont*, 31st biennial sess. (1931), no. 174, pp. 194–96.)

Notes

Notes to Introduction

1. Ernst Mayr, "The Origins of Human Ethics," in *Toward a New Philosophy of Biology: Observations of an Evolutionist* (Cambridge, Mass.: Harvard University Press, 1988), 80. Also see James F. Crow, "Eugenics: Must It Be a Dirty Word?" Review of *In the Name of Eugenics: Genetics and the Uses of Human Heredity*, by Daniel J. Kevles, *Contemporary Psychology* 33, no. 1 (Jan. 1988): 10–12.

2. Martin Pernick, "Eugenics and Public Health in American History," *American Journal of Public Health* 87, no. 11 (1997): 1767. For an excellent, accessible history of the eugenics movement and its legacy in current genetics research, see Diane B. Paul, *Controlling Human Heredity, 1865 to the Present* (Atlantic Highlands, N.J.: Humanities Press, 1995). For new perspectives on racism and eugenics, see Elazar Barkan, *The Retreat of Scientific Racism: Changing Concepts of Race in Britain and the United States between the World Wars* (Cambridge: Cambridge University Press, 1992). For recent historiographical trends, see Jonathan Harwood, "Genetics, Eugenics, and Evolution," *British Journal of the History of Science* 22 (1989): 257–65; Nils Roll-Hansen, "The Progress of Eugenics: Growth of Knowledge and Change of Ideology," *History of Science* 26, no. 73 (1988): 295–331; Garland E. Allen, "Eugenics and American Social History, 1880–1950," *Genome* 31, no. 2 (1989): 105–28.

3. For a comprehensive survey of eugenics leaders and organizations, see Barry Alan Mehler, "A History of the American Eugenics Society" (Ph.D. diss., University of Illinois, 1988).

4. David Starr Jordan, "The Eugenics of War: Its Effect Principally on Heredity, and Wholly Pernicious," *American Breeder's Magazine* 4, no. 3 (1913): 140–47; Theodore Roosevelt, "Twisted Eugenics," *Outlook* 106 (3 Jan. 1914): 30–34; Elazar Barkan, "Reevaluating Progressive Eugenics: Herbert Spencer Jennings and the 1924 Immigration Legislation," *Journal of the History of Biology* 24, (spring 1991): 91–112; Diane B. Paul, "Free Love and Birth Control," in *Controlling Human Heredity*, 91–96. For the penetration of eugenic ideology in American institutions, see Marout Arif Hasian Jr., *The Rhetoric of Eugenics in Anglo-American Thought* (Athens: University of Georgia Press, 1996).

5. See the following articles in *We Vermonters: Perspectives on the Past*, ed. Michael Sherman and Jennie Versteeg (Montpelier: Vermont Historical Society, 1991): Samuel B. Hand, "Stocking the State: Observations on Immigrants, Emigrants, and Those Who Stayed Behind," 95–106; T. D. Seymour Bassett, "Some Intolerant Vermonters," 135–44; D. Gregory Sanford, "A Hardy Race: Forging the Vermont

Identity," 341–47. Kevin Dann, "From Degeneration to Regeneration: The Eugenics Survey of Vermont, 1925–1936," *Vermont History* 59, no. 1 (1991): 5–29. Nazi themes are feature in Kevin Dann, "The Purification of Vermont," *Vermont Affairs* 4 (summer/fall 1987): 27–31; Michael Oatman, "Long Shadows: Henry Perkins and the Eugenics Survey of Vermont," exhibit at Robert Hull Fleming Museum, Burlington, Vt., fall 1995. James Bandler, "The Perkins Solution," *Sunday Rutland Herald*, 9 April 1995; "Facing Vermont's Dark Past," *Boston Sunday Globe* (3 Sept. 1995); Sally Pollak, "Pure Vermont," *Burlington Free Press* (17 Sept. 1995).

6. Charles Delaney and Christopher Roy, "Eugenics Genetics, Ethics and Art," symposium at Robert Hull Fleming Museum, 24 Oct. 1995; John Moody, "The Impact of Eugenics on Abenaki Familes in Vermont," New England American Studies Association, Providence, R.I., 27 April 1996; Charles Delaney, "Victims Left Out," *Burlington Free Press*, 4 Nov. 1995.

7. Barkan, *Retreat of Scientific Racism*, 269–73.

8. See, for example, Troy Duster, *Backdoor to Eugenics* (New York: Routledge, 1990); Lawrence Wright, *Twins and What They Tell Us about Who We Are* (New York: John Wiley, 1997); Carol Krause, *How Healthy Is Your Family Tree? A Complete Guide to Tracing Your Family's Medical and Behavioral History* (New York: Fireside, 1995); Jack C. Westman, M.D., *Licensing Parents: Can We Prevent Child Abuse and Neglect?* (New York: Insight Books, 1994). See particularly Westman, chapters 1, 2, 4, and 5, which link the cost and consequences of incompetent parenting of the "underclass" to the erosion of our quality of life.

Notes to Chapter 1

1. For two perspectives on George Perkins's career at UVM, see Kevin T. Dann, "The Natural Sciences and George Henry Perkins," in Robert V. Daniels, ed., *The University of Vermont: The First Two Hundred Years* (Hanover, N.H.: University Press of New England, 1991), 138–59; T. D. Seymour Bassett, "George H. Perkins," *A History of the Vermont Geological Surveys and State Surveyors* (Burlington: Vermont Geological Survey, 1976), 19–24.

2. For Dean Perkins's admiration for his son's generation, see George H. Perkins, "Fifty Years of College Leaves Teacher Optimist," *Vermont Alumni Weekly* 11 (4 April 1923), 1.

3. For the history of Christian Darwinism, see James R. Moore, *The Post-Darwinian Controversies: A Study of the Protestant Struggle to Come to Terms with Darwin in Great Britian and America, 1870–1900* (Cambridge: Cambridge University Press, 1979), 253–98. Moore discusses the philosophy of Asa Gray and George Frederick Wright, whose works George Perkins used in his teaching in addition to works that appear in Harry Perkins's library record.

4. Many sources confirm George Perkins's Christian Darwinism. In a resolution of appreciation for George Perkins the UVM trustees noted, "He was never able to discover any conflict between his science and religion, and instead found the teachings of science the strongest bulwark of his Christianity." See "Trustees of the University Express Their Regret and Appreciation," *Vermont Alumni Weekly* (4 Oct. 1933): 4.

5. For the popularity of Christian Darwinism at UVM, George Perkins's public commentary on evolution and its expression in his anthroplogy course in the 1890s, see Kevin Dann, "The Natural Sciences and George Henry Perkins," *The University of Vermont: The First Two Hundred Years*, ed. Robert V. Daniels (Hanover, N.H.: University Press of New England, 1991), 154.

6. Mrs. A. W. Slocum, 1929, typed MS., George H. Perkins papers, folder: "Perkins, Mary," UVM Archives, Burlington, Vermont; "Mary Farnham Perkins," obituary, *Burlington Free Press*, 11 May 1904. G. H. Perkins papers, "Perkins Family," UVM Archives.

7. Eagle Camp, organized in 1891, offered science summer programs for boys, girls, and eventually teachers. Concerning this and George Perkins's Vermont field excursions, see Bassett, "George H. Perkins," 18–22. For Harry Perkins's photographs of Vermont landscapes, see G. H. Perkins papers, UVM Archives.

8. Z. Philip Ambrose, "The Curriculum: I. From Traditional to Modern," in Daniels, *University of Vermont*, 100.

9. Ibid., 94–97.

10. University of Vermont, *The Catalogue of the University of Vermont and State Agricultural College*, 1896–1897 (Burlington: University of Vermont), 28–32 (hereafter cited as *UVM Catalogue*); T. D. Seymour Bassett, "The Classical College"; "President Matthew Buckham," in Daniels, *University of Vermont*, 81–82, 111–12.

11. George H. Perkins, "Fifty Years of College Teaching," 1–2.

12. The Founder's Day address, given by important alumni, celebrated the virtues of the humanistic, Congregationalist values embodied in the Marsh curriculum. T. D. Seymour Bassett, "A Small University with Ivy League Aspirations," in Daniels, *University of Vermont*, 32–33; J. Kevin Graffagnino, "A Hard Founding Father to Love," in Daniels, *University of Vermont*, 197–98.

13. "Kakewalker in '95, Prof. Henry Perkins Recalls Informality," *Burlington Free Press* (2 Feb. 1952), clipping, Faculty files, folder: "Henry F. Perkins," UVM Archives; James W. Loewen, "Black Image in White Vermont: The Origin, Meaning, and Abolition of Kake Walk," in Daniels, *University of Vermont*, 353.

14. UVM *Catalogue*, 1896–1897, 66; Faculty files, "Henry F. Perkins," UVM Archives.

15. This discussion of Brooks and his influence on Perkins is derived from three sources: Garland E. Allen, "The Morphological Tradition and W. K. Brooks," in *Thomas Hunt Morgan: The Man and His Science* (Princeton, N.J.: Princeton University Press, 1978), 35–46; Dennis M. McCullough, "W. K. Brooks's Role in the History of American Biology," *Journal of the History of Biology* 2 (1969): 411–38; and E. A. Andrews et al., "William Keith Brooks: A Sketch of His Life by Some of His Former Pupils and Associates," *Journal of Experimental Zoology* 9, no. 1 (1910): 1–52. The editorial board of this journal, which was made up of America's leading zoologists and Brooks's most eminent students, dedicated this volume to his memory "as a token of affection and respect."

16. Henry F. Perkins, "The Development of Gonionema Murbochii," *Proceedings of the Academy of Natural Sciences of Philadephia* 54 (Dec. 1902): 750–90. For Brooks's teaching, see McCullough, "W. K. Brooks's Role," 431.

17. McCullough, "W. K. Brooks's Role," 425–57. In the latter half of the nine-

teenth century, physiology (including biochemistry, microbiology, and related fields in medicine) and "biology," which then was synonymous with natural history, comprised two relatively autonomous fields of inquiry. Physiologists searched for mechanisms of life in laboratory experiments on cells and tissues and biochemical analysis. Natural historians were field biologists, whose laboratories were used to culture, dissect, observe, and carefully document the process of development and behavior under natural conditions. A realignment of these autonomous fields of the life sciences into experimental embryology, evolution, and heredity began in earnest around 1900, as a growing number of highly motivated biologists, dissatisfied with the speculative nature of natural history, were drawn to investigation of the mechanisms of heredity, growth, and development, which were being more fruitfully elucidated through advances in cell theory and experimental embryology. Perkins attended Johns Hopkins prior to its transition to the "experimental tradition" after 1910 and after the training of Brooks's most gifted students in the 1880s, who adopted some of the new methods and theories of German embryologists and physiologists. Garland G. Allen, *Life Science in the Twentieth Century* (New York: John Wiley, 1975), 2–9, 18–20, 21–39.

18. Otto C. Glaser, in "William Keith Brooks: A Sketch of His Life," 16–17. For Brooks's philosophy, see H. V. Wilson, "Writings on the Principles of Science," in "William Keith Brooks: A Sketch of His Life," 39–43.

19. For Brooks's changing views on heredity, see Allen, *Thomas Hunt Morgan*, 38–39; H. V. Wilson, in "William Keith Brooks: A Sketch of His Life," 37–39. For the origins of Weismann's theory and its importance in the defense of Darwinism, see Peter J. Bowler, *The Mendelian Revolution: The Emergence of Hereditarian Concepts in Modern Science and Society* (Baltimore: Johns Hopkins University Press, 1989), 83–92. For neo-Darwinians' refutations of Herbert Spencer's theories of evolutionary progress, see Peter J. Bowler, "The Role of the History of Science in the Understanding of Social Darwinism and Eugenics," *Impact of Science on Society* 40, no. 3 (1990): 273–78.

20. George Lefevre, in "William Keith Brooks: A Sketch of His Life," 13, 16. Diverse interpretations of heredity and evolution added to the political, scientific, and social ferment at the turn of the century. See Diane B. Paul, *Controlling Human Heredity, 1865 to the Present* (Atlantic Highlands, N.J.: Humanities Press, 1995), 30–42; Ronald W. Clark, *The Survival of Charles Darwin: A Biography of a Man and an Idea* (New York: Random House), 203–20.

21. Mendel's laws of heredity, for example, were rejected by neo-Darwinians because proponents refuted the Darwinian assertion that species developed from gradual modifications shaped by natural selection. They suggested that mutants or hybrids could form new species and imposed metaphysical explanations for the nature of "unit characters" (genes). Experimental embryologists also adopted neo-Lamarckian views, challenging Weismann's theory of the germplasm.

22. For some of his publications, see Faculty file, folder: "Henry F. Perkins," UVM Archives. Brooks and Perkins were in Dry Tortugas the summer of 1905. "Henry Farnham Perkins," *The Vermont Cynic* (29 May 1926); E. G. Conklin, in "William Keith Brooks: A Sketch of His Life," 24.

23. Henry F. Perkins to Charles B. Davenport, 2 May 1903. C. B. Davenport papers, American Philosophical Society (hereafter APS), Philadelphia.

24. Perkins's development of the zoology curriculum (1902–1923) is summarized in Nancy Gallagher, "Henry Farnham Perkins and the Eugenics Survey of Vermont" (master's thesis, University of Vermont, 1996, Appendix A, pp. 321–22).

25. Joseph A. Caron, "'Biology' in the Life Sciences: A Historiographical Contribution," *History of Science* 26, no. 73 (1988): 223–68. Library Circulation Records, Henry Perkins, 1902–1913, UVM Archives, 124–27, 317–24, 475–76, 479–80, 484–85, 37–38, 56. Harry Perkins's course descriptions appear consistent with advocates of similar approaches at Harvard and Johns Hopkins. For the role of neo-Darwinism within the scientific controversies of this period, see Allen, *Thomas Hunt Morgan*, 106–42; Peter J. Bowler, *Evolution: The History of an Idea* (Berkeley: University of California Press, 1989), 246–81; Bowler, *The Mendelian Revolution*, 110–38.

26. Thomson, *The Science of Life: An Outline of the History of Biology and Its Recent Advances* (Chicago: Herbert Stone, 1899), quotes in Preface, p. 162. Perkins had evidently not reached the conclusion of many American biologists that Mendel's laws had provided "the answer," for the first evidence of his interest in this new research appears in 1912.

27. Joseph McCabe, introduction to *Last Words on Evolution*, by Ernst Haeckel, trans. Joseph McCabe (London: A. Owen & Co.), 7–8.

28. Haeckel, *Last Words*, 96–111, quotes on pp. 101, 111.

29. Guy Potter Benton, "Inaugural Address," in Charles R. Cummings, "The Inauguration As I Saw It," *Vermonter* 16, no. 11 (Nov. 1911): 371–94, quote on p. 373.

30. Benton, "Inaugural Address," 377–80.

31. Ibid., 385–87.

32. Carnegie Foundation for the Advancement of Teaching, *A Study of Education in Vermont*, Bulletin no. 7 (New York: Carnegie Foundation, 1914), 8, 93; Guy P. Benton, quoted in Robert O. Sinclair, "Agricultural Education and Extension," in Robert V. Daniels, ed., *University of Vermont*, 188. For faculty responses to President Benton's initiatives, see T. D. S. Bassett, "Small University with Ivy Aspirations," 199–201.

33. The chromosome theory of heredity did not achieve completion and full recognition as verification of Mendelian genetics until 1915, with the landmark treatise, *The Mechanism of Mendelian Heredity* (New York: Henry Holt & Co., 1915) by T. H. Morgan, A. H. Sturtevant, H. J. Muller, and C. B. Bridges. Yet the Columbia team's Drosophila studies on mutations, sex determination, and chromosome mapping were published in journals and gaining rapid acceptance after 1910. See Allen, *Life Science in the Twentieth Century*, 56–65.

34. Perkins used zoology and embryology texts by Vernon Lyman Kellogg, David Starr Jordan, and William E. Kellicott. Kellicott lectured on eugenics in 1910; he published his lecture in *The Social Direction of Human Evolution: An Outline of the Science of Eugenics* (New York: Appleton, 1923). Kellogg and Jordan both published extensively on eugenics. Kellogg's studies of social insects became a point of departure for thinking about his topics "Inheritance of Mind," "Social Organization and Mental Capacity," "Racial Traits and Immigration," as well as discussion of race deterioration in the World War I draft broad tests, in *Mind and Heredity* (Princeton: Princeton University Press, 1923). Eugenic ideas were promoted in Kellogg's *Human Life as the Biologist Sees It* (New York: Holt, 1922) and *Evolution* (New York: Appleton, 1924).

35. Philip R. Reilly, *The Surgical Solution: A History of Involuntary Sterilization*

in the United States (Baltimore: Johns Hopkins University Press, 1991), 58–60. The committee, headed by New York attorney Bleeker Van Wagenen, was composed of physicians, with the exception of Harry Laughlin, director of the Eugenics Record Office, who served as its secretary. Notable consultants included Lewellys Barker of the Johns Hopkins School of Medicine, Henry Goddard, geneticist Raymond Pearl of the University of Michigan (later of Johns Hopkins), and Lewis Marshall, leader of the American Jewish Congress. For the first wave of sterilization laws, see Reilly, *Surgical Solution*, 41–55.

36. Genetics research in the United States received substantial support from the American Breeders' Association. Davenport established the Eugenics Record Office as an adjunct to the most highly funded biological enterprise in the United States, the Station for Experimental Evolution at Cold Spring Harbor. Davenport's research in human heredity was financed by Mrs. E. H. Harriman and the Carnegie Institution of Washington. The most complete history of the Eugenics Record Office is Garland E. Allen, "The Eugenics Record Office at Cold Spring Harbor, 1910–1940," *Osiris*, 2nd ser., 2 (1986): 225–64.

37. Other works by J. Arthur Thomson (and Geddes) included *Darwinism and Human Life*, and *Heredity* (New York: G. P. Putnam's Sons, 1908), *Evolution Theory* (London: E. Arnold, 1904), and *Evolution of Sex* (London: W. Scott, 1901). Interestingly, he did not borrow *Parasitism Organic and Social* (London: S. Sonnenschein, 1895). The only eugenics treatise in his library circulation records prior to 1913 was John B. Haycroft's *Darwinism and Race Progress* (London: Sonnenschein, 1895). Haycroft, in the Milroy lectures of 1894 to the Royal College of Physicians, lamented the rising incidence of feeblemindedness in the English race and promoted Francis Galton's 1890s version of eugenics. Haycroft advocated segregation in institutions of "incapables" and linked his argument to the rights of children and the obligations of parenthood, community responsibility, and education of the "masses" in matters of heredity and evolution. Perkins was thus acquainted with the British version of eugenics as early as 1906 and absorbed eugenics from a turn-of-the-century neo-Darwinian perspective rather than a Mendelian orientation.

38. J. Arthur Thomson, *Heredity*, 504, 506, 519.

39. Ibid., 274–75.

40. Ibid., 526–30.

41. Ibid., 305–6.

42. William Bateson (1905), quoted in Thomson, *Heredity*, 508.

43. Thomson, *Heredity*, 530. While Thomson may have been referring to surgical sterilization advanced by British physician Robert Reid Rentoul in *Race Culture or Race Suicide? A Plea for the Unborn* (London: Walter Scott, 1906), he more likely was referring to 'The Remedy" advanced by British physician W. Duncan McKim in *Heredity and Human Progress* (London: Stationer's Hall, 1899). McKim's "remedy" was a "gentle, painless death," an "expression of the enlightened pity for the poor victims . . . too defective in nature to find true happiness in life" (p. 188). Rentoul also discusses euthanasia, castratrion, decriminalization of attempted suicide, and abortion of fetuses of "lunatic" women. Thomson cited these works as examples of "Spartan" methods of eugenics (pp. 564, 572). Neither Rentoul nor McKim appear in Harry Perkins's library record.

44. Daniel J. Kevles, *In the Name of Eugenics* (Berkeley: University of California Press, 1985), 391. Perkins, like many other eugenists of the period (and some critics of mainline eugenics), advocated restriction of reproduction of social or mental "inferiors" based on interactionist views of heredity and environment.

45. *Vermont Bulletin*, 1911–1912, 143.

46. William Albert Locy, *Biology and Its Makers* (New York: H. Holt, 1908). This was an updated version of Thomson's *Science of Life*, emphasizing developments in experimental physiology and embryology, cell theory and the germ theory of disease, the theories of heredity of Mendel, Galton, and Weismann, and, of course, "The Rise of Evolutionary Thought." For course description, see *Vermont Bulletin*, 1913–1914, 157.

47. "Henry Farnham Perkins," *Vermont Cynic*, 29 May 1926; "Study of Lake Fish Begins," *Burlington Free Press*, 4 July 1913. Faculty file, "Henry F. Perkins," UVM Archives.

48. The title "Fellow by Courtesy" was considered an honor at Johns Hopkins reserved for only select scholars. His topic of research, "the problem of rhythmic activities in certain lower animals," suggests that he was hoping to update his research in the tradition of Herbert Jennings's work on the behavior of protozoa. See Kathryn Allamong to T. D. S. Bassett, 13 April 1973, Faculty files, "Henry F. Perkins," UVM Archives. Publications on descriptive zoology gave way after 1910 to experimental subjects, even in journals such as the *American Naturalist*. Allen, *Thomas Hunt Morgan*, 33–34, n. 11.

49. Dean Perkins acknowledged such a role for the new generation of professors. Modern college education, he contended, required a faculty of specialists who could adapt their teaching to broader social and cultural needs of society. G. H. Perkins, "Fifty Years of College," 1.

50. For a comprehensive analysis of the context, history, and problems with these tests, see Stephen J. Gould, "The Hereditarian Theory of I.Q.," in *The Mismeasure of Man* (New York: Norton, 1981), 146–233.

51. *UVM Bulletin*, 1919–1920, 130. Perkins's new course offerings were consistent the new realignment of "biology" into embryology, heredity, and evolution. Allen, *Life Science in the Twentieth Century*, 113–14.

52. In 1923, Perkins expanded the heredity course into two three-hour courses, Zoology 10 (Heredity) and Zoology 11 (Modern Theories of Evolution). He continued to teach embryology in the 1920s. *UVM Bulletin*, 1923–1924, 157. He added a separate course in eugenics (Zoology 12) in 1932, which was taught by his assistant, Elin Anderson (1932–1936).

53. Irving Lisman, personal interview, 15 Oct. 1995; Laura Bliss and Henry F. Perkins, "Fifteen Pairs of Twins: A Study of Similarities," *Eugenical News* 13 (1928): 92–93. Lisman took Perkins's heredity course in 1932. Laura Bliss used the twin study for her senior thesis. Perkins used his influence to secure its publication and promoted her efforts to secure a position at the Eugenics Record Office at Cold Spring Harbor. See Perkins to Davenport, 15 May 1928, C. B. Davenport papers, APS.

54. Horatio H. Newman, *Readings in Evolution, Genetics, and Eugenics* (Chicago: University of Chicago Press, 1921), viii.

55. The scientific legitimacy the theory enjoyed and the tenacity with which ge-

neticists supported Mendelian explanation for feeblemidedness are analyzed in David Barker, "The Biology of Stupidity: Genetics, Eugenics, and Mental Deficiency in the Inter-War Years," *British Journal of the History of Science* 22 (1989): 347–75.

56. Henry H. Goddard, *Feeblemindedness: Its Causes and Consequences* (New York: Macmillan, 1914), 4.

57. Karl Pearson, F.R.S., *Eugenics Laboratory Lecture Series: The Francis Galton Laboratory for National Eugenics* (London: Dulace, 1909), 18–19, 33–38. Pearson advanced the use of public institutions as eugenics laboratories and linked the need for children to be more intelligent, adaptable, and educated to the modern demands of complex, industrial societies.

58. Goddard, *Feeblemindedness*, 571.

59. Paul Popenoe and Roswell H. Johnson, "Eugenics and Euthenics," quoted in Newman, *Readings*, 487. Strong hereditarian views appear in "The Inheritance of Human Characters" by Elliott B. Downing of the University of Chicago and "Human Conservation," in H. E. Walter, *Genetics* (New York: Macmillan, 1913).

60. H. E. Walter, "Human Conservation," in Newman, *Readings*, 476. Some of the texts of the late 1920s cite Harry Laughlin's statistical studies of immigrants and debate their significance, discuss the multiple meanings of the term "race" and the myth of race purity, and stress that cultural heritage is as important to consider as biological heritage. See Michael F. Guyer, *Being Well-Born: An Introduction to Heredity and Eugenics* (Indianapolis: Bobbs-Merrill, 1927), 396–411. The anti-Semitic and anti-southern-European sentiment featured in traditional histories of the eugenics movement was not universal. See Elazar Barkan, "Reevaluating Progressive Eugenics: Herbert Spencer Jennings and the 1924 Immigration Legislation," *Journal of the History of Biology* 24, no. 1 (1991): 91–112.

61. Caleb Williams Saleeby, "The Promise of Race Culture," in Newman, *Readings*, 504.

62. Ibid., 509. In 1911 Perkins had read Saleeby's *Evolution: The Master Key, a Discussion of the Principles of Evolution as Illustrated in Atoms, Stars, Organic Species, Mind, Society, and Morals* (London: Harper, 1906). The convergence of Perkins's interests in neo-Darwinism, Christian missionary work, and theology appeared in 1912–1913 when 70 percent of his library acquisitions concerned these subjects. The evidence suggests that religious appeal was an important and heretofore overlooked factor in Perkins's participation in eugenics.

63. The Kallikaks were a New Jersey family. The Nams and Jukes were New York families and may have particularly interested Perkins for their proximity to Vermont. For analyses of the family studies and their influence, see Allen, "The Eugenics Record Office," 242–45; Paul, *Controlling Human Heredity*, 50–65; Nicole Hahn-Rafter, *White Trash: The Eugenic Family Studies, 1877–1919* (Boston: Northeastern University Press, 1988).

64. Dugdale and other nineteenth-century reformers' views rested on Lamarckian theories of soft heredity, which, they believed, education and rehabilitation could correct. See Paul, *Controlling Human Heredity*, 42–45, 49.

65. *UVM Bulletin*, 1921–1922, 136–38. The prerequisite for the social ethics course was Philosophy 2 (Ethics), which surveyed the "historical development of man's moral consciousness as he rises from savagery and advances to civilization," or

social psychology, both taught by Gifford. Psychology professor Metcalf taught psychological applications, a course in the nature and uses of mental testing.

66. H. F. Perkins to C. B. Davenport, 9 Feb. 1923; C. B. Davenport to H. F. Perkins, 13 Feb. 1923. C. B. Davenport papers, APS, Philadelphia.

67. H. F. Perkins, "A Resumé of an Eleven Years Study, 1925–1936," Guide to the Collection (ca. 1938), 1–2, Eugenics Survey of Vermont papers, Public Records Office, Middlesex, Vt. (Hereafter, ESV papers.)

68. C. B. Davenport to H. F. Perkins, 20 Feb. 1923, C. B. Davenport papers, APS, Philadelphia.

69. H. F. Perkins, "Resumé of an Eleven Years Study," 2.

70. Charles B. Davenport to Henry F. Perkins, 20 Feb. 1923. C. B. Davenport papers, APS, Philadelphia.

71. No manuscripts of Jennie Schneller's work have surfaced, yet she apparently alerted Perkins to some inconsistencies in the data. See H. F. Perkins to C. B. Davenport, 12 Mar. 1924 and 6 May 1925, C. B. Davenport papers, APS, Philadelphia. For Perkins's compilations of the draft board data and his lecture on their eugenic significance, see "Statistics—Federal Statistics of Draft Defects Found in Men Drafted in the World War," ESV papers.

72. H. F. Perkins, "Resumé of an Eleven Years Study," 1–2. The report to which Perkins referred was C. B. Davenport, "Defects Found in Drafted Men," *Scientific Monthly* (Jan. 1920): 5–25.

Notes to Chapter 2

1. For example, see Lydia Kingsmill Commander, *The American Idea* (New York: A. S. Barnes, 1907). Commander explored the range of opinion regarding the trend toward a small family and the contributing factors of changing women's roles, economic constraints, and higher expectations in rearing children. She developed the twin themes of immigration and the declining Anglo-American majority in her chapter, "Another Form of Race Suicide." For Theodore Roosevelt's promotion of eugenics, see Diane B. Paul, *Controlling Human Heredity: 1865 to the Present* (Atlantic Highlands, N.J.: Humanities Press, 1995), 100–105; Marouf A. Husian Jr., *The Rhetoric of Eugenics in Anglo-American Thought* (Athens: University of Georgia Press, 1996), 45–50.

2. Paul, *Controlling Human Heredity*, 97–100, 105; John M. Lund, "Vermont Nativism: William Paul Dillingham and the U.S. Immigration Legislation," *Vermont History* 63, no. 1 (1995): 15–29; Maudean Neill, *Fiery Crosses in the Green Mountains: The Story of the Ku Klux Klan in Vermont* (Randolph Center, Vt.: Greenhills Books, 1989).

3. For the influence of eugenics on American immigration laws, see Elazar Barkan, *The Retreat of Scientific Racism: Changing Concepts of Race in Britain and the United States between the World Wars* (Cambridge: Cambridge University Press, 1992), 66–76, 189–203; and "Reevaluating Progressive Eugenics: Herbert Spencer Jennings and the 1924 Immigration Legislation," *Journal of the History of Biology* 24, no. 1 (1991): 91–112; Garland E. Allen, "The Eugenics Record Office at Cold Spring

Harbor, 1910–1940," *Osiris*, 2nd ser. 2 (1986): 247–50; Philip R. Reilly, *The Surgical Solution: A History of Involuntary Sterilization in the United States* (Baltimore: Johns Hopkins University Press, 1991), 62–65.

4. Paul C. Dunham, *Population Trends and Their Implications on Government in Vermont* (Burlington: University of Vermont, Government Research Center, 1963), 2–6; Harold Fisher Wilson, *The Hill Country of Northern New England: Its Social and Economic History in the Nineteenth and Twentieth Centuries* (Montpelier: Vermont Historical Society, 1947), 369, 388–91. Samuel B. Hand, Jeffrey Marshal, and D. Gregory Sanford, "'Little Republics': The Structure of State Politics in Vermont, 1854–1920," *Vermont History* 53 (summer 1985): 145. More recent studies have challenged the rural migration "facts," yet census data of this nature was used by Harry Perkins and contemportaries. For other opinions see Kevin Dann, "From Degeneration to Regeneration: The Eugenics Survey of Vermont, 1925–1936," *Vermont History* 59, no. 1 (1991): 6–7; H. Nicholas Muller III, "From Ferment to Fatigue? 1870–1900: A New Look at the Neglected Winter of Vermont," Occasional Paper, (Burlington, Vt.: Center for Research on Vermont, 1984).

5. Rowland E. Robinson, *Vermont: A Study in Independence* (Boston: Houghton, Mifflin, 1892), 330. Robinson's narratives represent a revival of early nineteenth-century Vermont history writing that invoked frontier legends, made heroes of the Allen brothers and the Green Mountain boys in the Revolution and Vermont statehood, and celebrated the old Vermont stocks as uniquely patriotic, independent, and self-sacrificing. See Randolph Roth, "Why Are We Still Vermonters? Vermont's Identity Crisis andd the Founding of the Vermont Historical Society," *Vermont History* 59 (fall 1991): 197–211; Jeffrey P. Potash, "Deficiencies in Our Past," *Vermont History* 59 (fall 1991): 212–26. The myth that Native Americans (the Western Abenaki) had vacated Vermont in the seventeenth century persisted into the 1970s, despite evidence to the contrary. See William A. Haviland and Marjory W. Power, *The Original Vermonters: Native Inhabitants Past and Present* (Hanover, N.H.: University Press of New England, 1994), 2, 238–46.

6. Robinson, Vermont: A Study in Independence, 331.

7. Wilbert L. Anderson, *The Country Town: A Study of Rural Evolution* (1906; reprint New York: Arno Press, 1974), 168.

8. Charles Otis Gill, *The Country Church: The Decline of Its Influence and the Remedy* (New York: Macmillan, 1913) and Charles Gill and Gifford Pinchot, *Six Thousand Country Churches* (New York: Macmillan, 1920); Bibliography, Guide to the Collection of the Eugenics Survey, 238.

9. Wilson, *Hill Country of Northern New England*, 346–80. Between 1900 and 1930 one-fourth of all farms were given up and the land under cultivation declined by 34 percent. Property tax reform was not initiated until 1930. Wilson notes that these factors encouraged contemporaries to praise or condemn the farmer according to the value of his land, as either adaptable (good) or marginal and dispensable.

10. Liberty Hyde Bailey, *The Country Life Movement in the United States* (New York: Macmillan, 1911); William L. Bower, *The Country Life Movement in America, 1900–1920* (Port Washington, N.Y.: Kennikat, 1974).

11. Rebek, Andrea, "The Selling of Vermont: From Agriculture to Tourism, 1860–1910," *Vermont History* 44, no. 1 (1976): 14–27.

12. Dona L. Brown, *Inventing New England: Regional Tourism in the Nineteenth Century* (Washington, D.C.: Smithsonian Institution Press, 1995), chap. 5.

13. William Slade Jr., *Laws of Vermont, of a Public and Permanent Nature, Coming Down to, and Including, the Year 1825* (Windsor, Vt.: Simon Ide, 1825, for the State of Vermont), 370: quoted directly from Stephan R. Hoffbeck, "'Remember the Poor' (*Galatians* 2:10): Poor Farms in Vermont," *Vermont History* 57, no. 4 (fall 1989), 227.

14. Hoffbeck, "'Remember the Poor,'" 229–230; Alden M. Rollins, *Vermont Warnings Out* (Camden, Me.: Picton Press, 1995), 1–23. Rollins's four volumes list all the "warnings out" in Vermont in the early nineteenth century. Many of the family names that appear in these volumes also appear in the "Special Pedigees" of the Eugenics Survey.

15. Orphanages and foster home placement organizations gradually replaced apprenticeships and "binding out" orphans or abandoned children after the Civil War. Such arrangements provided care for healthy, well-behaved children. See Lorenzo D'Agostino, *The History of Public Welfare in Vermont* (Winooski, Vt.: St. Michael's College Press, 1948), 131–38; L. Josephine Webster, *The Vermont Children's Aid Society, Inc.: The First Fifteen Years, 1919–1934,* (Burlington, Vt.: Queen City Printers, 1964), 21–22.

16. D'Agostino, *History of Public Welfare*, 133–34, 252–57.

17. *The Annual Report of the Home for Destitute Children* (Burlington, Vt.: R. S. Styles, 1893), 10. The home was founded in 1865 for homeless and destitute children by a group of civic-minded, middle-class Burlington women. Concentration of French Canadian and Irish immigrants in tenements; concern that Burlington, as a lake port, was becoming a "city of the transient poor"; and anxiety over the "vice, filth, and poverty" they associated with these developments contributed to their desire to provide poor children with such a refuge. See Marshall True, "Middle Class Women and Civic Improvement in Burlington, 1865–1890," *Vermont History* 56, no. 2 (1988): 112–27. Harry Perkins's mother served on the board of directors of the HDC from 1894 until her death in 1904, during Harry's formative years.

18. Sarah Torrey, *Annual Report of the Home for Destitute Children* (Burlington, Vt.: R. S. Styles, 1899), 8–9; Torrey, *Annual Report* (1895), 13–14.

19. Torrey, *Annual Report of the Home for Destitute Children* (1897), 10–11. For context of Torrey's remark, see James W. Trent, *Inventing the Feeble Mind: A History of Mental Retardation in the United States* (Berkeley: University of California Press, 1994), 79–88. The American developments between the 1880s and 1930s that Trent describes were experienced in Vermont as well, only telescoped into roughly a fifteen-year period (1915–1930).

20. The increased demand for use of this facility was in part the result of increasing the age of eligible persons. See D'Agostino, *History of Public Welfare*, 215.

21. Vermont, General Assembly, *Journal of the Senate of the State of Vermont* (Monpelier: State of Vermont, 1913), 618–21.

22. Reilly, *Surgical Solution*, 30–55. Opponents of sterilization argued that sterilization of defectives would lead to licentiousness and the spread of venereal disease, that the claims of the therapeutic benefits were doubtful, or that such a procedure was unconstitutional, beyond the powers of the state. With the notable exception of Franz

Boas, there was surprisingly little discussion over the accuracy of medical diagnosis of mental defect or its alleged hereditary origins.

23. "Scope of the Conference," *Proceedings of the Vermont State Conference of Charities and Corrections* (Montpelier, Vt.: The Conference, 1916), 1; W. J. Van Patten, "President's Address," *Proceedings of the Vermont Conference of Charities and Corrections* (1917), 4. (Hereafter *Proceedings VCCC.*)

24. K. R. B. Flint, *Poor Relief in Vermont* (Northfield, Vt.: Norwich University Studies, 1916).

25. Ibid., 7–9.

26. *General Laws of Vermont*, Act chap. 319, 92, 1915 (Montpelier: State of Vermont, 1917), 1242.

27. Ibid.

28. W. J. Van Patten, "The Children of Vermont: Provisions Made by the State for the Dependent, Neglected, and Delinquent Children of the State," *Proceedings of the VCCC* (1917), 36.

29. Ibid., 40.

30. Webster, *Vermont Children's Aid Society*, 13–14.

31. *General Laws of Vermont*, title 42, chap. 319, 1917.

32. K. R. B. Flint, "Vermont Conditions and Needs," *Proceedings VCCC* (1917), 11–12.

33. W. H. Jeffrey, "The Work of the Board of Charities and Probation," *Proceedings of the Third Annual Vermont Conference of Social Work* (Montpelier, Vt.: The Conference, 1918): 6 (hereafter *Proceedings VCSW*).

34. Ibid., 9–10.

35. Charles Dalton, "Public Health Service," *Proceedings VCSW* (1918), 27–36. Also see Charles Caverly, M.D., "The Needy Child: From the Viewpoint of the State Board of Health," *Proceedings VCCC* (1917), 21–23. For an overview of the relationships between eugenics and public health, see Martin S. Pernick, "Eugenics and Public Health in American History," *American Journal of Public Health* 87, no. 11 (1997): 1767–72.

36. Webster, *Vermont Children's Aid Society*, 22.

37. Michael Sherman, "'Spanish Influenza' in Vermont 1918–1919" (paper presented to the Research-in-Progress Seminar, Center for Research on Vermont, University of Vermont, 13 October 1993).

38. Webster, *Vermont Children's Aid Society*, 9–13.

39. Ibid., 86: "By-Laws of the Vermont Children's Aid Society, Inc.," Article 2: "Purpose."

40. Webster, *Vermont Children's Aid Society*, 28. Vermont looked to the "Massachussetts Plan" of a census as its model; the Vermont Conference of Social Work (VCSW) and the Vermont Children's Aid Society (VCAS) relied heavily on consultants from public and private agencies in Massachussetts. See, for example, C. C. Carstens, "A Militant Plan of Child Welfare Work," *Proceedings VCCC* (1917), 14–15; and Robert W. Kelso, Massachussetts Commissioner of Public Welfare, "The Unmarried Mother," *Proceedings VCSW* (1920), 21–26. Henry W. Thurston, head of the Department of Child Welfare at the New York School of Social Work, helped the Vermont Children's Aid Society define its mission.

41. Webster, *Vermont Children's Aid Society*, 78–80.

42. Ibid., 26. Webster cited a case in which a judge was hesitant to commit a child to an unknown organization until he saw the list of directors, some of whom he knew by reputation at least. He responded, "Anything they stand for is OK with me." The *Burlington Free Press* article (2 April 1919) is reproduced in Webster, 10–12.

43. Ibid., 25. Sara Smart, "The Social Exchange," *Proceedings VCSW* (1920), 35–37. Central indexes of the so-called 3 D's date back to the 1880s and were inspired by Frederick Wines's survey of the 1880 census and its report, *The Defective, Dependent, and Delinquent Classes of the United States* (Washington, D.C.: Government Printing Office, 1881). See Trent, *Inventing the Feeble Mind*, 77–79. The Indiana Central Index, for example, listed over 40,000 persons in 1920. Indiana was the first state to pass a sterilization law and its index provided information for extensive eugenics studies on particular families. The National Conference of Charities and Correction spearheaded the promotion of state indexes. For its development in Indiana, see Amos W. Butler, "Some Families as Factors in Anti-Social Conditions," in *Eugenics, Genetics, and the Family*, vol. 1, *Scientific Papers of the International Congress of Eugenics*, ed. Charles B. Davenport et al. (Baltimore: Williams & Wilkins, 1923), 387–97.

44. Webster, *Vermont Children's Aid Society*, 50–51. Before 1925 there was no minimum marriage age if the parents consented. The minimum age in 1925 for minors (14 for girls and 16 for boys) was raised in 1929 to 16 for girls and 18 for boys.

45. L. Josephine Webster, "Report of the General Secretary," *VCAS Second Annual Report* (Oct. 1921), 11–12.

46. Ibid., 9–12; Harriett E. Abbott, "True Stories of Vermont Women," *VCAS First Annual Report* (Oct. 1920), 23–27; L. Josephine Webster, "Child Wives," *VCAS Ninth Annual Report* (Oct. 1928), 16. Abbott's and Webster's efforts to place potentially "sex-delinquent" young women in institutions reflected a larger national trend in social work. See Mary E. Odem, *Delinquent Daughters: Protecting and Policing Female Sexuality in the United States, 1885–1920* (Chapel Hill: University of North Carolina Press, 1995).

47. A. R. Gifford, "Report of the President," *VCAS Second Annual Report* (Oct. 1921), 23–24.

48. W. H. Jeffrey, "State Work for Children," *Proceedings VCSW* (1920), 52.

49. Hand, Marshall, and Sanford, "'Little Republics,'" 152–54.

50. Paul C. Dunham, *Vermont State Administrative Agencies*, (Burlington: University of Vermont Government Research Center, 1965), 48–49.

51. Ibid., 78–80, 87–90.

52. L. Josephine Webster, "The Work of the Children's Aid Society," *Proceedings VCSW* (Oct. 1920): 46–47. Also see Flint, "Vermont Conditions and Needs," 13.

53. By 1925 the VCAS cases had swelled to 520, and many remained untouched. See Webster, *Vermont Children's Aid Society*, 31–33. For problems of feebleminded children, see Webster, *Vermont Children's Aid Society*, 40–47; and *VCAS Sixth Annual Report* (1925), 10–11; Jeffrey, "State Work for Children," 54; T. J. Allen, "New Opportunities for the Feebleminded in Colonies," *Proceedings VCSW* (1925), 7. Agitation for a state census of the feebleminded continued throughout the 1930s, until the state finally agreed to one in 1942. See Margaret B. Whittlesey, *The Vermont Conference of Social Welfare: The First Fifty Years, 1916–1966* (Burlington: VCSW, 1966), 8–11.

54. For efforts to expand mental testing, see Webster, *Vermont Children's Aid Society*, 38, 44–45; "Proposals for Social Legislation," *Proceedings VCSW* (1925), 13–15. For Abbott's training at the Eugenics Record Office, see Davenport to Perkins, 14 May 1925, C. B. Davenport papers, American Philosophical Society, Philadelphia.

55. L. Josephine Webster, "Report of the General Secretary," *VCAS Sixth Annual Report* (Oct. 1925), 7–13; quotation on p. 7.

56. For more information on the Eugenics Survey benefactors, see Dann, "From Degeneration to Regeneration," 8; Catherine Ashburner, "Shirley Farr" in *Those Intriguing, Indomitable Vermont Women* (U.S.: Vermont State Division of AAUW, 1980), 41–42; G. W. Bailey to Perkins, 28 May 1934. Guy W. Bailey papers, folder: H. F. Perkins, 1934, UVM Archives.

57. Webster, "Report of the General Secretary," *VCAS Sixth Annual Report* (1925), 13. Perkins's own agenda was more specific. While negotiating for Harriett Abbott's services, he confided to Charles Davenport that the necessary family data had "already been corralled, and made up in graphic form . . . just waiting to be whipped into shape and checked up from original resources." He had the "promise of editorial support from most of the state newspapers" for a campaign for sterilization. Perkins to Davenport, 6 May 1925, C. B. Davenport papers, APS, Philadelphia.

Notes to Chapter 3

1. Minutes of the first Advisory Committee Meeting of the Eugenics Survey of Vermont (hereafter ESV), 26 Sept. 1925; Perkins to Advisory Committee, 4 Sept. 1925, Advisory Committee, ESV papers. For Perkins's proposed plan, see Truman Allen file, Paul Moody papers, Box 181, UVM Archives, Burlington, Vt. (hereafter reference to this file is cited as Allen file, Moody papers).

2. Minutes of the first Advisory Committee Meeting of the ESV, 26 Sept. 1925; Perkins to Advisory Committee, Sept. 1925, Advisory Committee, ESV papers.

3. Roy Lubove, *The Professional Altruist: The Emergence of Social Work as a Career, 1880–1930* (New York: Atheneum, 1975), 55–83, 109–114; James W. Trent, *Inventing the Feeble Mind: A History of Mental Retardation in the United States* (Berkeley: University of California Press, 1994), 154–92. Most historians present the eugenics and mental hygiene movements as separate and theoreticallly antagonistic, yet Perkins's dovetailing of the two approaches demonstrates the potential compatibility of eugenics and new trends in psychiatry.

4. *Report of the Annual Meeting of the Vermont Conference of Social Work* (Montpelier, Vt.: The Conference, 1925), 7–9 (hereafter VCSW, *Report of Annual Meeting*); Perkins to Advisory Committee, Sept. 1925, Advisory Committee, ESV papers.

5. Lubove, *Professional Altruist*, 40–49, 140–44.

6. For a description of the training program for social workers in eugenics at the Eugenics Record Office, see Amy Sue Bix, "Experiences and Voices of Eugenics Field Workers: 'Womens Work' in Biology," *Social Studies of Science* 27 (1997): 625–68. Garland E. Allen, "The Eugenics Record Office at Cold Spring Harbor, 1910–1940," *Osiris* 2nd series 2 (1985), 239–242.

7. H. F. Perkins to T. J. Allen, 16 Jan. 1926, Allen file, Moody papers.

8. William J. Robinson, M.D., *Woman: Her Sex and Love Life* (New York: 1917; reprint, Eugenics Publishing Co., 1927); Bibliography, Guide to the Collection, 240, ESV papers. Abbott relied on a variety of contemporary sources in mental hygiene and psychology as well. Her understanding of feeblemindedness relied on these sources and her own well-worn copy of Florence M. Teagarden, *A Study of the Upper Limits of Intelligence* (New York: Teachers' College, Columbia University, 1924), more than on her training at the Eugenics Record Office. See Books and Monographs, ESV Papers.

9. H. F. Perkins, "A Resumé of an Eleven Years Study, 1925–1936," Guide to the Collection (ca. 1938), 5, ESV papers.

10. Perkins to Advisory Committee, 12 Oct., 1926; VCSW, *Report of Annual Meeting* (1926 and 1927). For Perkins's initial publicity of the ESV work, see H. F. Perkins, "Summary of the Family Tree Charts Underway on May 17, 1926" in "Statistics: Federal Statistics of Draft Defects," ESV papers; H. F. Perkins, "Progress in the Survey of the Feebleminded," VCSW, *Report of Annual Meeting* (1926), 10; H. F. Perkins, "Review of Eugenics in Vermont," *Vermont Review* (Sept.–Oct. 1926): 56–59; Perkins's address to the Women's Auxillary to the Dairymen, "Heredity Is Big Problem," *Burlington Free Press*, 29 Oct. 1926.

11. H. F. Perkins to Members of the Advisory Committee, 22 Oct. 1926, Allen file, Moody papers; Minutes of the ESV Advisory Committee Meeting, 28 Oct. 1926; Perkins to Horace G. Ripley (Brattleboro Retreat), 2 Nov., 1926, Advisory Committee, ESV papers. For the historical context of Dr. Allen's concerns, see Trent, *Inventing the Feeble Mind*, 198–201.

12. Asa Gifford, Vermont Conference of Social Work Committee on Legislation, *Proposals for Improving Social Legislation in Vermont* (1 Jan. 1927), 7, Vermont Conference of Social Work, ESV papers.

13. Roswell Johnson to H. F. Perkins, 15 Jan. 1927; Perkins to Johnson, 21 Jan. 1927, American Eugenics Society Papers, American Philosophical Society, Philadelphia.

14. Arthur H. Estabrook, "The Tribe of Ishmael," in *Eugenics, Genetics, and the Family*: vol. 1, *Scientific Papers of the Second International Congress of Eugenics*, 1921, ed. Charles B. Davenport (Baltimore: Williams & Wilkins, 1923), 398–404. Estabrook's point of departure on the "Ishmael" family was the Rev. Oscar C. McCullough's paper on the Indiana Ishmaelites, read at the National Conference of Charities and Corrections at Buffalo in 1888. Estabrook used the expanding "central index" in Indiana to trace these kinship networks. "Nomadism," a compulsion to wander, had been studied and presented in eugenics literature as most likely caused by a recessive gene. See William J. Tinkle, "Heredity of Habitual Wandering," *Journal of Heredity* 18 (1927): 548–51.

15. Estabrook, "Tribe of Ishmael," 404.

16. H. F. Perkins, "Review of Eugenics in Vermont," 59; H. F. Perkins, *Lessons from a Eugenical Survey of Vermont: First Annual Report* (Burlington: Eugenics Survey of Vermont, 1927), 8.

17. Kevin Dann, "Gypsies in Vermont?" (paper presented at Warren Sussman Memorial Graduate History Conference, Piscataway, N.J., 7 April 1990); J. Kevin Graffagnino, "Arcadia in New England: Divergent Visions of a Changing Vermont,

1850–1920," in *Celebrating Vermont: Myths and Realities* (Hanover, N.H.: Unversity Press of New England, 1991), 53–54.

18. Gifford, *Proposals for Improving Social Legislation*, 4–5. Perkins's portrayal of the Abenaki families as wanderers of French Canadian origin simply restated an old myth in Vermont history writing dating back to Ira Allen. See John Moody, "The Native American Legacy," *Always in Season: Folk Art and Traditional Culture in Vermont*, ed. June C. Beck (Montpelier: Vermont Council on the Arts, 1982), 54–64; John Moody, "The Impact of Eugenics on Abenaki Families in Vermont" (Providence, R.I.: New England American Studies Association, 1996); William A. Haviland and Marjory W. Power, *The Original Vermonters: Native Inhabitants Past and Present* (Hanover, N.H.: University Press of New England, 1994), 242–55; Molly Walsh, "Vermont's Abenaki," *Burlington Free Press* 7 Jan. 1996.

19. Perkins, *Lessons*, 9.

20. Kevin Dann, "The 'Pirate Family'" (lecture presented at Robert Hull Fleming Museum, Burlington, Vt., Oct. 1994).

21. Perkins, *Lessons*, 8.

22. Ibid., 10–11.

23. Ibid., 16–17.

24. VCSW, *Report of Annual Meeting* (1927), 6; Perkins to Allen, 15 March 1927, Allen file, Moody papers. For Gifford's comments, see VCSW, *Report of Annual Meeting* (1928), 14.

25. *Buck v. Bell*, 274 U. S. 200 (1927); Philip P. Reilly, *The Surgical Solution: A History of Involuntary Sterilization in the United States* (Baltimore: Johns Hopkins University Press, 1991), 87–93.

26. T. J. Allen to H. F. Perkins, 2 Nov. 1926; H. F. Perkins to T. J. Allen, 5 Nov. 1926, Allen file, Moody papers.

27. Perkins to ESV Advisory Committee, 23 May 1927, Allen file, Moody papers. For Perkins's initial overtures to the U.S. Department of Agriculture, see Dann, "From Degeration to Regeneration," 17.

28. VCSW, *Report of Annual Meeting* (1927), 3–8; Report of Meeting of the Advisory Committee of the ESV, 5 Nov. 1927, G. W. Bailey papers, UVM Archives. For Josephine Webster's concern over publicizing negative conditions, see "Report of the General Secretary," *VCAS Seventh Annual Report* (Oct. 1926), 15.

29. See for example, Raymond Pearl, "The Biology of Superiority," *American Mercury* 1 (1927): 257–66.

30. Eugenics Survey of Vermont, *Second Annual Report of the Eugenics Survey of Vermont* (Burlington: The Survey, 1928), 4.

31. Ibid., 11.

32. See, for example, Wilhelmine E. Key, *Heredity and Social Fitness: A Study of Differential Mating in a Pennsylvania Family* (Washington, D.C.: Carnegie Institute of Washington, 1920).

33. Harriett E. Abbott, "An Expensive Luxury," *Second Annual Report of the Eugenics Survey of Vermont*, 17.

34. Ibid., 17–18.

35. Ibid., 15–16.

36. Harriett Abbott's correspondence, Special Pedigrees Complete-II, ESV papers.

37. For more on Taylor and an additional perspective on the VCCL, see Dann, "From Degeneration to Regeneration," 18–25. For contemporaries' perspectives, see Henry C. Taylor, "The Vermont Commission on Country Life," *Journal of Farm Economics* 12 (Jan. 1930); H. F. Perkins, "The Comprehensive Survey of Rural Vermont," *New England's Prospect* (New York: Special Publication no. 16 American Geographical Society, 1933): 206–12.

38. H. F. Perkins, "Suggestions from Dr. Estabrook", Jan. 1928, Personal Interviews, VCCL prior to 1931, ESV Papers.

39. H. F. Perkins, "A Comprehensive Rural Survey of Vermont," History of the Survey, VCCL prior to 1931; Report of First VCCL Executive Committee Meeting, 18 May 1928, VCCL Meetings (1928),VCCL prior to 1931, ESV papers.

40. H. F. Perkins, "The Comprehensive Survey of Rural Vermont," Address before the Episcopal Clergy of Vermont, Rock Point, 14 Sept. 1928, VCCL Addresses, VCCL prior to 1931, ESV papers.

41. Perkins to Truman Allen, 6 June 1927. Perkins wanted a physician or a psychologist with a Ph.D. who was qualified in mental testing and diagnosis of mental deficiency or illness. Perkins to Allen, 4 Aug. 1928, Allen file, Moody papers.

42. Perkins to Advisory Committee, 29 Aug. 1928; Report of the Annual Meeting of the Advisory Committee, 18 Oct. 1928; Advisory Committee, ESV papers. Analysis of the tourism agenda within the ESV town and key family studies lies beyong the scope of this study, but pertient sources may be found in "Towns Suggested for Study and Key Family Study," 1929, ESV papers. For connections between tourist appeal and uplifting Vermonters to a "higher level of life," see Henry C. Taylor, "The Vermont Commission on Country Life," VSCW, *Report of Annual Meeting* (1928), 8–9. Perkins's synthesis of eugenics and sociology was inspired by the research and advice of geographers Ellsworth Huntington of Yale and Goldthwait of Dartmouth. See James Walter Goldthwait, "A Town That Has Gone Downhill," *Geographical Review* 17 (Oct. 1927): 528–52; H. F. Perkins, Interview with Ellsworth Huntington, 25 May 1928, Personal Interviews, VCCL prior to 1931, ESV papers.

43. O. C. Cook, "Human Hybrids in Virginia," review of *Mongrel Virginians: The Win Tribe*, by Arthur H. Estabrook and Ivan E. MacDougle, *Journal of Heredity* 19 (Mar. 1928): 115–18.

44. H. F. Perkins to C. B. Davenport, 17 April 1928; C. B. Davenport to Perkins, 19 April 1928; Perkins to Davenport, 27 April 1928; C. B. Davenport papers, APS, Philadelphia. Perkins's request came on the heels of of a complaint from Carnegie Institution president John C. Merriam about the prejudice in Harry Laughlin's studies on immigration. For Davenport, this was the beginning of a growing dissatifaction with the scientific quality and propagandistic nature of eugenics activity at Cold Spring Harbor. See Reilly, *Surgical Solution*, 68–69; Garland E. Allen, "The Eugenics Record Office at Cold Spring Harbor, 250–51. For Perkins's research plan, see Nancy L. Gallagher, "Henry Farnham Perkins and the Eugenics Survey of Vermont" (Master's thesis, University of Vermont, 1996), 323–24.

45. Perkins to Davenport, 30 Dec. 1928; Davenport to Perkins, 31 Dec. 1928, C. B. Davenport papers, APS, Philadelphia.

46. Laura Bliss's consolation prize was publication of a brief article on her twin studies. Perkins to Davenport, 5 April 1928, 17 April 1928, 15 May 1928, C. B. Daven-

port papers, APS, Philadelphia; Laura P. Bliss and Henry F. Perkins, "Fifteen Pairs of Twins: A Study of Similarities," *Eugenics* 2, no. 2 (Feb. 1929): 22–26.

47. H. F. Perkins to C. B. Davenport, 5 Jan. 1929, C. B. Davenport papers, APS, Philadelphia. While it is tempting to speculate that Perkins was really in search of Native American ancestry among the French Canadians, Perkins would no doubt have been more explicit to Davenport of such suspicions if they existed and would have been quite boastful of such a "discovery."

48. Davenport to Perkins, 15 Jan. 1929, C. B. Davenport papers, APS, Philadelphia.

49. H. F. Perkins to C. B. Davenport, 17 Jan. 1929, C. B. Davenport papers, APS, Philadelphia.

50. Perkins had received a draft of the report and most of the statistics in 1927. The NCMH charts showing "native" and "foreign" inmates at Brandon Training School showed that the latter were in fact underrepresented at Brandon. Despite the fact that the survey of schoolchildren was conducted in predominantly "Yankee" towns, Vermont-born mothers had contributed a higher proportion of their offspring to the "subnormal" group than had mothers of foreign extraction. For the Brandon Training School report, see Allen file, Moody papers.

51. Davenport to Perkins, 21 Jan. 1929, 1 April 1929, and 15 April 1929, C. B. Davenport papers, APS, Philadelphia. In April, Davenport wrote to Perkins encouraging him to contact Estabrook, who was now available and would probably be interested in the French Canadian study. The letter was returned unanswered. Perkins solicited funds from Vermont business leaders in the granite, marble, and slate industries for research on racial questions, but the documents do not reveal Perkins's actual plans for their use. See Personal Interview with R. L. Patrick, Rock of Ages Co., 17 May 1929, Personal Interviews, VCCL prior to 1931, ESV papers.

52. Davenport and his associate, Morris Steggerda, attempted to demonstrate the inferiority of offspring from racially mixed marriages. Condemned by colleagues as scientifically flawed and highly prejudiced, the study became a lightning rod for controversies concerning biological definitions of race. Elazar Barkan, *The Retreat of Scientific Racism: Changing Concepts of Race in Britain and the United States between the World Wars* (Cambridge: Cambridge University Press, 1992), 162–68.

53. The study of "racial derivations and population problems" in the VCCL Committee on the Human Factor was delegated to Vassar professor Genieve Lamson, who would investigate population shifts and substitutions of old Vermont stock with immigrants as a demographic problem. See H. C. Taylor, "Annual Report of the Director to the Executive Committee of the VCCL" (1929), Annual Reports, VCCL prior to 1931, ESV papers.

54. H. F. Perkins to Dr. T. J. Allen, 4 Jan. 1929, Allen file, Moody papers.

55. With this decision, Perkins clarified his position against the pretentious role the Eugenics Record Office had suggested that Perkins assume in Vermont, that of a ruling body for the state on sterilization cases based on family history. See Laughlin to Abbott, 24 Sept. and 8 Oct. 1925, Miscellaneous: Letters of Special Interest, ESV papers.

56. Perkins to Advisory Committee, 13 Feb. 1929, G. W. Bailey papers, UVM Archives.

57. The Eugenics Survey of Vermont, *The Third Annual Report of the Eugenics Survey of Vermont* (Burlington: The Survey, 1929), 3.

58. Ibid., 4.

59. Henry F. Perkins and Francis E. Conklin, "The Children of Feebleminded and Insane Parents," *Third Annual Report of the Eugenics Survey of Vermont*, 14–16; "Children of Feebleminded and Insane Parents in the Pedigrees," Guide to the Eugenics Survey of Vermont Papers, 72–77, ESV papers.

60. *Third Annual Report of the Eugenics Survey of Vermont*, 7. "Unsocial" traits or "defects" included reputation for being "crazy," "low-grade" or extremely peculiar, low living standards evidenced by "dirty" homes and meager circumstances, insanity, deliquency, dependency, and "sex offenders."

61. Ibid., 10. The Rectors, like the Pirates, Doolittles, and Gypsies, were one of the original ten most intensively studied families. Abbott and Conklin's summary reports of 1927–1928 did not cast them in such a favorable light. This shows the flexibility with which the family data could be exploited for "public education" depending on the political climate or the particular agenda.

62. Ibid.

63. Ibid., 19.

64. Eugenics Survey of Vermont, "The Furman Family," *Third Annual Report of the Eugenics Survey of Vermont*, 20–24.

65. Eugenics Survey of Vermont, *Fourth Annual Report of the Eugenics Survey of Vermont* (Burlington: The Survey, 1930), 41–44; "Key Family Study: Lincoln," ESV papers. The *Fourth Annual Report* continued with these themes in their study of Williston ("Dunnfield") in "Changes in an Old Town and Some of Its Oldest Families," 24–29; Key Family Study: Williston, ESV papers.

66. Perkins to Guy W. Bailey, 1 July 1929, G. W. Bailey papers, UVM Archives. The threefold program of the Human Factor Committee would survey Vermont family life, population trends, and care of the handicapped.

67. This generalization oversimplifies a period of transition (ca. 1929–1933) in eugenics history, in which the vast and growing scholarship on its complexities, debates, and general ferment defy any simple categorizations. My purpose is to situate Perkins's work within this transistional context (Elazar Barkan's "lacuna," Daniel Kevles's transition from "mainline to reformed," and Garland Allen's shift from "old" to "new" eugenics). The ESV library shows Perkins's familiarity with the new research that defined the paradigm shift. His speeches and reports interpret Vermont's human resource concerns according to the idea that human diversity, like agricultural diversity, was a more scientific approach to eugenics. See O. F. Cook, "Quenching Life on the Farm: How the Neglect of Eugenics Subverts Agriculture and Destroys Civilization," review of *These Changing Times: A Story of Farm Progress during the First Quarter of the Twentieth Century*, by E. R. Eastman, *Journal of Heredity* 19 (Oct. 1928): 440–52.

68. Perkins declined the American Eugenics Society's offer to help him organize better-family contests or eugenics exhibits at state fairs, claiming the "time was not ripe" for such ventures in Vermont, and it was unfair to "[rub] it into a community that such conditions exist [degenerate families]" without solutions. They had also decided to "mark time here in Vermont" on the matter of sterilization. See Perkins to W. C.

Palmer, American Eugenics Society, 27 May 1930, American Eugenics Society Correspondence, ESV papers. For the appeal of Whitney's ideas in Kansas, see Laura Lovett, *Speaking in the Vernacular: Florence Sherbon and the Promotion of the Family Ideal, 1915–1935* (Indianapolis: Organization of American Historians, 1998).

69. "Psychological Tests at the Riverside Reformatory," Riverside Reformatory—Reports, ESV papers.

70. Eugenics Survey of Vermont, "Study of a Group of Women at Rutland Reformatory," *Fourth Annual Report*, 5–16.

71. Riverside Reformatory Study, ESV papers. Historian Hal Goldman's study of court cases in four Vermont counties has documented a dramatic escalation of prosecutions and convictions for adultery between 1880 and 1920 (interview by author with Hal Goldman, University of Massachussetts, September 1998). Women convicted of adultery continued to make up a large portion of the prison population during the interwar years.

72. Eugenics Survey of Vermont, *Fourth Annual Report*, 11.

73. Ibid., 10–11.

74. How many women in the Rutland Reformatory, prior to or after the passage of the sterilization law, were offered the option of an elective salpingectomy is unknown. If Vermont physicians followed the California model, many women may have been strongly encouraged to forgo future motherhood, perhaps as a condition for parole or as part of "the treatment needed to prepare them for reassuming the responsibilities and social standards demanded of its members by any community." See ESV, *Fourth Annual Report*, 7.

75. Martha M. Wadman to Supt. T. J. Allen, 29 July 1929, Allen file, Moody papers. Elin Anderson, Wadman's successor, took over the Brandon waiting list and was especially adamant about interviewing the individuals and their families. Perkins to Members of the Advisory Committee, 13 Jan. 1930, Allen file, Moody papers. For the context of Wadman's and Anderson's work, see Lubove, *Professional Altruist*, 108–14.

76. Eugenics Survey of Vermont, "Study of Waiting List for State School for Feebleminded," *Fourth Annual Report*, 16–20.

77. Ibid., 5.

78. Ibid., 36–40.

79. Ibid. The environmental thrust of eugenics, reflected in Perkins's "eugenical-sociological" studies, is also discussed in J. H. Kempton, "Heredity, Environment and Human Fate," review of *The Biological Basis of Human Nature* by Herbert S. Jennings, *Journal of Heredity* 21 (June 1930): 248–52; Paul Popenoe, "Feeblemindedness Today: A Review of Some Recent Publications on the Subject," *Journal of Heredity* 21 (Oct. 1930): 421–31.

80. William E. Castle to H. F. Perkins, 28 Mar. 1930. G. W. Bailey papers, UVM Archives, 1929–1930. Castle's revised views on race and heredity (which coincided with his praise of the Eugenics Survey) are discussed in Barkan, *Retreat of Scientific Racism*, 143–46.

81. Perkins to Advisory Committee, 10 Dec. 1929, Allen file, Moody papers.

82. Lubove, *Professional Altruist*, 113–14, 173–79.

83. For Perkins's praise of Anderson and the community philosophy, see Perkins, "Resumé of an Eleven Years Study," 18, 24–25. For her commitment to the commu-

nity philosophy, see Elin Lilja Anderson, *Rural Health and Social Policy* (Washington, D.C.: Michael M. Davis et al.), 1951.

84. Towns Suggested for Study—Information About Towns: Cornwall, Waitsfield, and Jamaica, ESV papers.

85. Elin J. Anderson, *Selective Migration from Three Rural Vermont Towns and Its Significance* (Burlington: Eugenics Survey of Vermont, 1931); Genieve Lamson, *A Study of Agricultural Populations in Selected Vermont Towns, 1929–1930* (Burlington: VCCL, 1931). The complete records of Anderson's migration study, including all interviews, are found in Migration Study, ESV papers.

86. Anderson, *Selective Migration*, 38.

87. Ibid., 63–66.

88. Ibid., 21–23, 66–69.

89. Ibid., 13–16, 69–73; VCCL Committee on Land Utilization, *Rural Vermont: A Program for the Future* (Burlington: VCCL, 1931), 148.

90. Henry C. Taylor, "Introduction," in VCCL, *Rural Vermont*, 1–5.

91. Committee on the Human Factor, "The People of Vermont," in VCCL, *Rural Vermont*, 11.

92. Ibid., 10–33.

93. Subcommittee on the Care of the Handicapped, in VCCL, *Rural Vermont*, 282–99.

94. Ibid., 288–89; Cheney C. Jones, "Needed Developments in Child Welfare in the Next Decade," VCSW, *Report of Annual Meeting* (1931), 17.

95. H. F. Perkins, "Eugenic Aspects," in VCCL, *Rural Vermont*, 300.

96. Ibid., 299–304.

97. Committee on Educational Facilities for Rural People, in VCCL, *Rural Vermont*, 278–79. Charles H. Dempsey, executive secretary of the Committee on Educational Facilities and commissioner of the Department of Education, also served on the ESV advisory committee throughout its existence.

98. William L. Bower, *The Country Life Movement in America* (Port Washington, N.Y.: Kennikat Press, 1974), 82–84. The Institute for Social and Religious Research was an official sponsor of the VCCL and conducted portions of the religion survey. For their survey data and reports, see VCCL Committee on Religious Forces, ESV papers.

99. Committee on Religious Forces, "Religious Forces," in VCCL, *Rural Vermont*, 348–70; the ESV and VCCL papers document favorable attitudes toward French Canadian Catholics who participated in community efforts and a suspicion of priests who discouraged such activity. Perkins, too, was impressed with French Candians like the ones in Whiting, Vermont, who helped to paint the Protestant church since it was the only church in town. "To my mind rather remarkable are the efforts of the community spirit in these French Canadians . . . their interest was solely that of community welfare." H. F. Perkins, Interview with A. M. Kelsey, Whiting, Vermont, 11 Dec. 1928, Personal Interviews, VCCL prior to 1931, ESV papers.

100. Committee on Religious Forces, "Religious Forces," in VCCL, *Rural Vermont*, 355–57.

101. Ibid., 367. For a discussion of Catholic opposition to eugenics and the pope's 1930 encyclical, see Reilly, *Surgical Solution*, 118–22.

102. Committee on the Conservation of Vermont Traditions and Ideals, "The Conservation of Traditions and Ideals," in VCCL, *Rural Vermont*, 371–85; Sara Cleghorn, "Coming Vermont: A Pageant," Pageant, VCCL prior to 1931, ESV papers; Dorothy Canfield Fisher, *Vermont Tradition: The Biography of an Outlook on Life* (Boston: Little, Brown, 1953). Fisher's elitist views as exposed in her writings on Vermont have attracted attention and controversy. For two different perspectives, see Hal Goldman, "'A Desirable Class of People': The Leadership of the Green Mountain Club and Social Exclusivity, 1920–1936," *Vermont History* 65 (summer/fall 1997), 137–41; Ida H. Washington, "Dorothy Canfield Fisher's *Tourists Accommodated* and Her Other Promotions of Vermont," *Vermont History* 65 (summer/fall 1997), 153–64.

103. H. C. Taylor, "Introduction," in VCCL, *Rural Vermont*, 1; W. H. Dyer to Perkins, 2 Feb. 1931, American Eugenics Society: Requests for Financial Assistance, ESV papers.

104. In 1930, Perkins began the national promotion of the VCCL as a model rural eugenics progam. His veiled sarcasm directed toward Davenport's lack of support is striking in Henry F. Perkins, "Rural Factors in Rural Communities," *Eugenics* 3, no. 8 (1930). For his promotion of the VCCL as a national model in eugenics, see H. F. Perkins, "An Experiment in Eugenics in Vermont," p. 5, Adult Education in Eugenics, ESV papers.

105. The rationale for sterilization in 1931 reflected a general shift in medical opinion. See Reilly, *Surgical Solution*, 89–93, 122–25; Trent, *Inventing the Feeble Mind*, 198–223.

106. H. F. Perkins to Marion Hansell, American Eugenics Society, 2 Jan. 1931, American Eugenics Society papers, APS, Philadelphia.

107. See newspaper clippings on sterilization, Henry F. Perkins, Faculty file, UVM Archives, Burlington, Vt.

108. *Laws of Vermont*, 31st biennial sess. (1931): No. 174—"An Act for Human Betterment by Voluntary Sterilization," 194–96. The senate passed the bill 22 to 8. The house voted 140 in favor and 75 opposed, winning by the same margin that defeated it in 1927. The Catholic Daughters of America at Waterbury were the first to officially oppose the bill when it was introduced in the house. See *Vermont House Journal*, 19 March 1931, p. 619. The legislature made two amendments to the original bill. It restricted fees of surgeons and physicians paid by the state and removed clauses authorizing overseers of the poor to arrange for sterilizations. See Report of the Committee on Public Health, Bill S. 64, 1931, Vermont State Archives, Montpelier.

Notes to Chapter 4

1. Perkins to Eugenics Survey of Vermont (hereafter ESV) Advisory Committee, 20 Jan. 1931; Minutes, ESV Advisory Committee, 15 Sept. 1931; Minutes, Joint Meeting of ESV and VCCL, 3 Dec. 1931; General file: Advisory Committee, ESV papers.

2. Minutes of the Board of Directors, American Eugenics Society, 3 April, 6 May, and 25 May 1931, American Eugenics Society (hereafter AES) papers, American Philosophical Society (hereafter APS), Philadelphia.

3. Frederick Osborn, "History of the American Eugenics Society," *Social Biology* 21, no. 2 (1974): 118; Osborne to Perkins, 18 Aug. 1931, American Eugenics Society Correspondence, ESV papers; Barry Alan Mehler, "A History of the American Eugenics Society" (Ph.D. diss., University of Illinois, 1988), 97–110. Documentation of favorable responses to the ESV annual reports may be found in Annual Reports, ESV papers.

4. Both Harry Laughlin and Clarence G. Campbell, director of the Eugenics Research Association at Cold Spring Harbor, resigned from the society in June 1931. Perkins was nominated to fill the vacancy left by geneticist Leslie C. Dunn, who refused his nomination to the board of directors. Cytologist Edwin G. Conklin had resigned from the AES board of directors the month before. AES minutes, 3 April 1931; 6 May 1931, 7 Oct. 1931, AES papers, APS.

5. Perkins's correspondence documents the AES crisis and his deliberations with the eugenics leadership. See AES Correspondence and Eugenics Research Association Correspondence, particulary correspondence between Perkins and Paul Popenoe and Edwin Gosney of the Human Betterment Foundation in California, ESV papers. For the controversies over birth control, see Roswell H. Johnson, "The Pope and Eugenics: A Reply to the Encyclical," *People* 1 (April 1931): 5–9, Pamphlet library, ESV papers; E. S. Gosney and P. Popenoe to Perkins, 22 April 1932, AES Correspondence, ESV papers.

6. Minutes, Meeting of the Board of Directors of the AES, 4 June 1932, AES papers, APS. Perkins was also unanimously elected at this meeting to serve as president of the society for the next three years.

7. Osborn later declared himself leader of the AES's repudiation of the Cold Spring Harbor group and publicized his refusal in 1940 of back copies of *Eugenical News* that contained Laughlin's pro-Nazi commentaries. In 1932 he had confidentially donated $100 to Perkins's effort to salvage the foundering AES by distributing copies of *Eugenical News* to 350 AES members. Fred Osborn to H. F. Perkins, 22 Sept. 1932, Finances, AES, ESV papers.

8. Osborn, "History of the American Eugenics Society," 118–19. In 1932, Perkins circulated a position statement, for the approval of the AES board of directors, supporting the legalization of birth control. Free access to contraceptives and birth control information was eugenic, he argued, because it would enable responsible, educated young adults to marry earlier without the fear of unplanned pregnancies and the resulting financial burdens. Research had shown that couples who married in their early twenties were better adjusted to married life, created a happier homes for children, and ultimately had larger families with an earlier start. Perkins to AES Board of Directors, 5 Dec. 1932, Birth Control Correspondence, ESV papers. Perkins had addressed the Birth Control League in Boston in 1931 and corresponded with Mararet Sanger, whose views on the subject evidently impressed him. Ellsworth Huntington and Henry Pratt Fairchild, Perkins's closest friends within the inner circle, strongly supported birth control as well.

9. "Immigration and Eugenics" with Gifford's annotations, 20 Jan. 1931, Advisory Committee; Leon Whitney to Perkins, Nov. 1930, Miscellaneous: American Eugenics Society, ESV papers; Minutes, AES board of directors meeting, 3 April 1931 and 21 Dec. 1932, AES papers, APS.

10. H. F. Perkins, "The Eugenics Survey of Vermont," paper and discussion at the Joint Session of the AES and the Eugenics Research Association, 4 June 1932, AES papers, APS, Philadelphia. For reviews of Anderson's migration study, see R. C. Cook, "Population Trends in Vermont," *Journal of Heredity* 23 (Mar. 1932): 131–34; Bessie Bloom Wessel, "Review of Eugenics Survey Report," *American Journal of Sociology* (Mar. 1932): 846–47; F. Osborne to Perkins, 21 Feb. 1933, AES Correspondence, ESV papers. For other responses and requests for ESV publications, see Annual Reports, ESV papers.

11. H. F. Perkins, "Contributory Factors in Eugenics in a Rural State," in *A Decade of Progress in Eugenics: Scientific Papers of the Third International Congress of Eugenics*, ed. Henry F. Perkins et al. (Baltimore: Williams & Wilkins, 1934), 183.

12. Ibid., 187. In the 1930s Perkins defended the enduring vigor of the old Vermont stocks, claiming that rural depletion in Vermont had not been harmful and that the "fine steady yeoman" still remains. See "Looks to Rural Life to Preserve Race," *New York Times*, 5 June 1932, 29.

13. Ibid., 188. For a photograph of Perkins's exhibit, see Eugenics Congress, ESV papers. The original of the pedigree chart is stored in the UVM Archives; Perkins's other charts remain in private hands.

14. A. W. Forbes, "Is Eugenics Dead?" *Journal of Heredity* 24 (April 1933): 143.

15. Leon Whitney, "Neither Dead nor Sleeping"; H. R. Hunt, "Interest Increasing"; C. C. Little, "Not Dead but Sleeping," *Journal of Heredity* 24 (April 1933): 149–51.

16. C. G. Campbell, "The Present Position of Eugenics," *Journal of Heredity* 24 (April 1933): 144–47.

17. H. F. Perkins, "Make Haste Slowly," *Journal of Heredity* 24 (April 1933): 148.

18. Ibid., 148–49. Perkins noted that the recent sterilization laws were more sound than the early laws and only succeeded after a "vigorous campaign of education."

19. Perkins to Advisory Committee, April 1932; 31 Mar. 1933. General file: Advisory Committee, ESV papers; Elin Anderson, Summary of Findings, Institute on "Helping People in Need," in *Report of the Annual Meeting of the Vermont Conference of Social Work* (Montpelier: The Conference, 1933) (hereafter VCSW, *Report of Annual Meeting*). For Perkins's contributions, see H. F. Perkins, "Radio Series on *Rural Vermont: A Program for the Future*," 5 Nov. 1932, and "Human Aspects of Biology: Address to the State Teachers Association Convention," Dr. Perkins' Speeches, ESV papers. For twin research, see Adoption Study, ESV papers; Marion Baldwin, "A Study of Three Pairs of Identical Twins with Reference to Their Comparative Abilities in Various Motor and Mental Tests," (Master's thesis, University of Vermont, 1930).

20. Bessie Bloom Wessel, *An Ethnic Survey of Woonsocket, Rhode Island* (Chicago: University of Chicago Press, 1931); Christine Avghi Galitzi, *A Study of Assimilation among Roumanians in the United States* (New York: Columbia University Press, 1929). Galitzi's insightful discussion of theories of racial integrity, assimilation and Americanization is essential to understanding the intellectual context of Anderson's work. Galitzi's argument for importance of immigrant influence in the enrichment and development of American life permeates Anderson's interpretations of the ethnic study (pp. 156–72). Racist Madison Grant's *The Alien in Our Midst* (1930) and Harry

Laughlin's controversial immigrant studies were also in the ESV library, but they evidently did not serve as models for Anderson's ethnic study.

21. Robert S. Lynd and Helen Merrell Lynd, *Middletown: A Study in Contemporary Culture* (New York: Harcourt, Brace, 1929) and *Middletown in Transition: A Study in Cultural Conflicts* (New York: Harcourt, Brace, 1937). Clark Wissler, whom Perkins consulted for his French Canadian Study, may have been the common denominator in these associations, for Wissler wrote the introductions to the Woonsocket survey and *Middletown*. Yet Wessel was familiar with Anderson's work, and Asa Gifford was using *Middletown* in his sociology classes.

22. Perkins to Advisory Committee, 31 March 1933, Advisory Committee, ESV papers.

23. In Germany, compulsory sterilization was decided by Hereditary Health Courts for persons diagnosed with "congenital feeblemindedness," schizophrenia, manic-depressive insanity, hereditary epilepsy, Huntington's chorea, hereditary blindness and deafness, severe physical deformities, and alcoholism. The German law, inspired by the California law and Harry Laughlin's model sterilization law, required physicians and public health officials to report any such cases they encountered in the general population during the course of their professional duties. See Reilly, *The Surgical Solution* (Baltimore: Johns Hopkins University Press, 1991), 105–10; Paul Popenoe, "The German Sterilization Law," *Journal of Heredity* 25 (July 1934): 257–60. For the synthesis of racism, eugenics, and anti-Semitism in Nazi eugenics and its relationships with Anglo-American eugenics, see Henry Friedlander, *The Origins of Nazi Genocide: From Euthanasia to the Final Solution* (Chapel Hill: University of North Carolina Press, 1995), 9–35; Fritz Lenz, "Eugenics in Germany," *Journal of Heredity* 15, no. 3 (1924): 223–31; Gotz Aly, Peter Chroust, and Christian Pross, *Cleansing the Fatherland: Nazi Medicine and Racial Hygiene*, trans. Belinda Cooper (Baltimore: Johns Hopkins University Press, 1994), 14–17, 156–62; Stefan Kuhl, *The Nazi Connection: Eugenics, American Racism, and German National Socialism* (New York: Oxford University Press, 1994).

24. Gypsies, for example, were arrested as criminals or "asocials" and studied and sterilized before they were classified by race scientists as inferior and later killed for that reason. Feeblemindedness also was loosely applied, as it had been in the United States. See Friedlander, *Origins of Nazi Genocide*, 21–35.

25. Paul Popenoe, Annual Report of the Human Betterment Foundation (13 Feb. 1934), Human Betterment Foundation, ESV papers.

26. H. H. Goddard to Perkins, 27 Jan. 1934, Financial Assistance Requests, ESV papers.

27. Goddard's Bureau of Juvenile Research was established to investigate and rule on all cases of suspected mental defect among Ohio's dependent and delinquent youth. Unlike Perkins, Goddard was an outsider and imposed his authority on child welfare workers and superintendents of county detention centers, often in direct conflict with their own programs for dependent children. The Division of Child Welfare resented his intrusion, rejected his methods, and ultimately brought down his organization. Goddard abandoned his effort to incarcerate Ohio's "feebleminded" in 1922 in order to teach psychology at Ohio State University. See Patrick J. Ryan, "Unnatural Selection: Intelligence Testing, Eugenics, and American Political Cultures,"

Journal of Social History 30, no. 3 (1997): 669–85. For Goddard's recantment, see Kevles, *In the Name of Eugenics* (Berkeley: University of California Press, 1985), 148–49, 206–7.

28. Perkins to Goddard, 1 Feb. 1934, Financial Assistance Requests, ESV papers.

29. In June 1933, Perkins had consulted Huntington over a proposal made by Guy Irving Burch, director of the Population Reference Bureau in Washington, D.C., to enlist support for eugenics among patriotic organizations such as the American Legion, the Federation of Labor, and the Chamber of Commerce by emphasizing its relevance to immigration. Huntington responded, "[H]is suggestion of getting tied up with the American Legion does not appeal to me. If the Eugenics Society is to do its best work I think it must remain aloof from the organizations which show a racial prejudice. We ought to make it clear to all the world that we are just as much interested in a high-grade Italian or a high-grade Chinese as in a high-grade Anglo-Saxon . . . the practical effect of getting tied up with the American Legion or some of the patriotic societies might be to make people think that we belong to the Nordic boosters." Perkins agreed, and discouraged Burch from making those sorts of connections. Guy Irving Burch to H. F. Perkins, 30 May 1933; Perkins to Huntington, 3 June 1933; Huntington to Perkins, 17 June 1933; Perkins to Huntington, 26 June 1933, Ellsworth Huntington papers, Manuscripts and Archives, Yale University Library, New Haven, Conn.; Perkins to Burch, 26 June 1933, AES Correspondence, ESV papers. For revision of the catechism, see Perkins to Huntington, 26 Dec. 1933, Huntington papers, Yale University Library, New Haven; Osborn, "History of the American Eugenics Society," 118–19. For ESV funding difficulties, see Perkins to Ellsworth Huntington, 26 April 1933, AES Correspondence, ESV papers; Perkins to Advisory Committee, 25 May 1934, Advisory Committee, ESV papers.

30. Perkins to Ellsworth Huntington, 26 April 1933, Ellsworth Huntington papers, Manuscripts and Archives, Yale University Library, New Haven; Paul Popenoe to Perkins, 4 May 1933, AES Correspondence, ESV papers.

31. Leon F. Whitney to Perkins, 15 Jan. 1934, AES Correspondence, ESV papers.

32. Elin Anderson, Interviews: Germans, Jewish, Yankees, Irish, 1933, Ethnic Study, ESV papers.

33. For Perkins's illness and colleagues' response, see Minutes, AES Board of Directors Meeting, 15 Feb. 1934, AES papers, APS, Philadelphia; Henry Pratt Fairchild to Harry Perkins, 26 April 1934, AES Correspondence, ESV papers. For his sabbatical plans, see Perkins to G. W. Bailey, 26 Jan. 1933; 26 Jan. 1934, G. W. Bailey papers, UVM Archives.

34. Perkins, "Make Haste Slowly," 149.

35. Perkins to ESV Advisory Committee, 25 May 1934, Advisory Committee, ESV papers; "Professor Perkins and Family to Tour Europe," *UVM Alumni Weekly*, 10 Nov. 1934, UVM Archives; Clarence G. Campbell, "The Biological Foundations of Our Social Philosophy," Presidential Address, Annual Meeting of the Eugenics Research Association, New York City, 2 June 1934, *Eugenical News* 20, no. 2 (1935): 17–25.

36. Mixed responses to the German Sterilization Law and the Myerson Report are extensively documented in primary and secondary sources. See for example, Reilly, *Surgical Solution*, 108–10, 122–26; P. Popenoe, Reports to the Board of Direc-

tors of the Human Betterment Foundation, 13 Feb. 1934, 12 Feb. 1935, 11 Feb. 1936, Human Betterment Foundation, Family Relations, ESV papers. For influential studies in England, see Kevles, *In the Name of Eugenics*, 148–63. German Hereditary Health Courts ordered the sterilization of nearly 60,000 persons in 1934, inspiring renewed campaigns for sterilization laws in America and abroad and a more powerful response by opponents. Sterilization laws passed in South Carolina (1935) and Georgia (1937), for example, but failed to override the governor's veto in the Alabama legislature, in part due to the organized religious opposition warning of "Hitlerizing" Alabama. See Edward J. Larsen, *Sex, Race, and Science: Eugenics in the Deep South* (Baltimore: Johns Hopkins University Press, 1995), 125–53. For successful campaigns for sterilization, see Nils Roll Hansen, "Eugenic Sterilization: A Preliminary Comparison of the Scandanavian Experience to That of Germany," *Genome* 31, no. 2 (1989): 890–95; and "Baltic Eugenics" *Journal of Heredity* 29, no. 3 (1938): 99–100.

37. J. H. Kempton, "Sterilization for Ten Million Americans," review of Leon F. Whitney, *The Case for Sterilization* (New York: Frederick Stokes & Co., 1934), *Journal of Heredity* 25 (Oct. 1934): 415–18. Whitney proved his detractors correct with this final piece of propaganda. Not only did it display his lack of understanding of genetics and changing attitudes on sterilization, but his reputed lack of academic integrity became obvious when he quoted on the book cover, under the heading "To the Author," 1928 letters from scientists to the AES praising eugenics. Vermont had no official agency, like the Bureau of Juvenile Research in California or eugenics boards in departments of public welfare of other states, to identify or research the backgrounds of candidates for sterilization. What role the Eugenics Survey played (perhaps unofficially) in specific sterilization cases is not documented in the ESV archive.

38. H. J. Muller (1890–1967) is known to biologists for his work with mutations and for his contributions to understanding the mechanism of gene action. As a member of Thomas Hunt Morgan's research team at Columbia (1912–1920), he made important contributions to the chromosome theory of heredity and was awarded the Nobel Prize for his 1927 discovery of the influence of radiation on the rate of mutations in Drosophila. See Garland Allen, *Thomas Hunt Morgan: The Man and His Science* (Princeton, N.J.: Princeton University Pres, 1978), 169–79; E. A. Carlson, "H. J. Muller," *Genetics* 70 (1972): 1–30.

39. H. J. Muller, *Out of the Night: A Biologist's View of the Future* (New York: Vanguard Press, 1935; reprint, New York: Garland Publishing Col., 1985), preface. Many historians continue to accept Mark Haller's interpretation of Muller's position as representing biologists' disenchantment with eugenics, "which ceased to be regarded as a science by the 1930s and was not so much opposed as ignored." Mark H. Haller, *Eugenics: Hereditarian Attitudes in American Thought* (New Brunswick, N.J.: Rutgers University Press, 1963), 169, 183. For a critical reassessment of the historiogaphy, see Nils Roll-Hansen, "The Progress of Eugenics: Growth of Knowledge and Change of Ideology," *History of Science* 26, no. 73 (1988): 295–331.

40. Muller, *Out of the Night*, 113.

41. For Muller's Marxist assault on capitalistic eugenics at the Third International Congress of Eugenics in 1932, see H. J. Muller, "The Dominance of Economics over Eugenics," in *A Decade of Progress in Eugenics: Scientific Papers of the Third International Congress of Eugenics*, ed. Harry F. Perkins et al. (Baltimore: Williams &

Wilkins, 1934), 138–44. Debates over the politics of eugenics are documented in the *Journal of Heredity* during the years 1936–1939. For "Bolshevik eugenics" and socialists' support for eugenics, see Diane Paul, "Eugenics and the Left," *Journal of the History of Ideas* 45 (Oct.–Dec. 1984): 567–90. For Muller's professional isolation due to his politics, see Kevles, *In the Name of Eugenics*, 186–92.

42. For Huxley's reversal of his views on race and eugenics, see Elazar Barkan, *Retreat of Scientific Racism*, 228–48, 296–310. For his promotion of eugenics in the United States in the 1930s, see J. H. Huxley, "The Vital Importance of Eugenics," *Harpers* 163 (Aug. 1931): 324–31; "Huxley Envisages the Eugenic Race," *New York Times*, 6 Sept. 1937, 19.

43. Julian S. Huxley and A. C. Haddon, *We Europeans: A Survey of "Racial" Problems* (London: Jonathan Cape, 1935), 7.

44. Ibid., 8.

45. Ibid., 107–9. Eventually, such statistical methods were developed and inspired a multitude of studies on racial differences, most recently surfacing in Richard J. Herrnstein and Charles Murray, *The Bell Curve: Intelligence and Class Structure in American Life* (New York: Free Press, 1994).

46. Huntington to Perkins, 10 Sept. 1935. AES Correspondence, ESV papers.

47. Ellsworth Huntington and the Directors of the American Eugenics Society, *Tomorrow's Children: The Goal of Eugenics* (New York: John Wiley & Sons, 1935), vii. Henry F. Perkins is one of the directors. Whitney had been replaced by a new executive director of the AES just prior to Perkins's resignation as president in 1934.

48. Ibid., 9.

49. Ibid., 31.

50. Ibid., 95.

51. Ibid., 35–36.

52. Huntington nevertheless advocated sterilization for individuals with severe disabilities, including "feeblemindedness," or for potential parents who are "carriers of recessive traits which ruin the happiness of their children." Ibid., 53.

53. Ibid., 58. Huntington noted that the depression of 1929–1934 had probably inhibited responsible couples from having children and that economic reforms would engender confidence in the future. For the eugenics of rural improvement, see ibid., 76–81.

54. Ibid., 68–70.

55. Ibid., 45–46.

56. Ibid., 103–14.

57. See, for example, S. J. Holmes, "'Facts of Heredity' for Race Conscious Germany," review of *Erblehre und Rassenhygiene im Volkischen Staat*, ed. Ernst Rudin, 1934, *Journal of Heredity* 25 (Oct. 1934): 418–20.

58. "Environment in a Eugenics Program: Dr. Julian Huxley See[s] Joint 'Nature-Nurture' Attack Necessary," editorial, *Journal of Heredity* 27 (Aug. 1936): 314–17; Robert Cook, "A Eugenics Program," *Journal of Heredity* 27 (April 1936): 195–200. Cook, a eugenicist himself, had criticized the race rhetoric, unsubstantiated scientific claims, and religiosity of 1920s eugenics propaganda. For the acceptance of the AES revision as the antithesis of Nazism and racism, see Clarette P. Armstrong, "Toward a Democratic Eugenics: A Review of *American Eugenics Today*," *Journal of Heredity* 30 (April 1939): 163–65.

59. *American Eugenics Today*, a pamphlet published in 1939 by the directors of the AES (which included Harry Perkins), summarized these revisions. Frederick Osborn expanded the idea of a "democratic" eugenics in his own books, *Preface to Eugenics* (New York: Harper & Bros., 1940, 1951) and *The Future of Human Heredity: An Introduction to Eugenics in Modern Society* (New York: Weybright & Talley, 1968). Osborn successfully convinced historians that he alone led the revolt against the "old eugenics" and the conversion of the AES, a myth that persists in most eugenics scholarship today. For more critical interpretations of Osborn's role, see Barkan, *Retreat of Scientific Racism*, 268–76, 328–32; Mehler, "History of the American Eugenics Society," 111–27.

60. Osborn had nominated Perkins to the Eugenics Research Association executive board in 1932 as part of the plan to merge with the AES and to heal the schisms within American eugenics. See Perkins to C. G. Campbell, 8 June 1932, AES Correspondence, ESV papers. For Campbell's and Laughlin's pro-Nazi sentiments and the consequences see "Praise to Nazis," *Time* 26 (9 Sept. 1935): 20–21; Allen, "The Eugenics Record Office at Cold Spring Harbor," 251–53; Kevles, *In the Name of Eugenics*, 355, n. 18.

61. The assassination of the Austrian prime minister Englebert Dollfuss by Nazi supporters and Mussolini's deployment of troops on the Italian border to check Nazi aggression just prior to the Perkinses' departure for Europe may have discouraged him from taking his family into those countries. Perkins returned from his sabbatical with publications from French and English eugenics societies for the Eugenics Survey library and requested Huntington to send a copy of *Tomorrow's Children* to a Parisian eugenicist, Mme Berti Albrecht. Henry F. Perkins, Faculty Information Card, 4 Nov. 1935, Faculty files, UVM Archives; Perkins to Huntington, 9 Oct. 1935, AES Correspondence, ESV papers. Also see French eugenics publications, "Le Problem Sexuel," ESV Pamphlet Library. For Perkins's fund-raising efforts with Shirley Farr, the Social Science Research Council, and the Milbank Foundation, see Bailey to Perkins, 29 Oct. 1935; Perkins to Bailey, 4 Nov. 1935, G. W. Bailey papers, UVM Archives; Perkins, Interviews with Donald Young and Frank Notestein, Sept. 1935, Interviews, ESV papers.

62. Max Hall, *Harvard University Press: A History* (Cambridge, Mass.: Harvard University Press, 1986), 68, 76. For the title, see p. 221 n. 33; Perkins to Huntington, 8 Jan., 19 Feb. 1936, AES Correspondence, ESV papers.

63. Anderson, *We Americans*, 3–4.

64. Ibid., 5–6.

65. Ibid., 18–19.

66. Ibid., 22.

67. Ibid., 8.

68. Ibid., 15.

69. Ibid., xii, 21–24.

70. Ibid., 29–30; Anderson, interview notes, "Dr. Perkins re. French Canadians," Interviews: French Canadians, Ethnic Study, ESV papers.

71. Anderson, *We Americans*, 29.

72. Ibid., 255.

73. Ibid., 28.

74. Ibid., 226–27.

75. Ibid., 30.

76. Ibid., 64.

77. Ibid., 263.

78. Ibid., 222.

79. Ibid., 237–38.

80. Ibid., 237, 241–42.

81. Ibid., 242–43. Interview with Fr. Parizo, Fr. Desautels, 8 Nov. 1933, General Interviews; Interview with Mr. Cate, YMCA, 20 Nov. 1933, Interviews: Yankees, Ethnic Study, ESV papers.

82. Anderson, *We Americans*, 241; E. Anderson, interview with I. Kiely, 11 Nov. 1933, Interviews—Irish; Interview with Mrs. Mildram, City Charity Dept., 1933, Interviews: Yankees, Ethnic Study, ESV papers..

83. Anderson, *We Americans*, 222–44, quotation on p. 244.

84. Regarding sterilization, see Anderson, *We Americans*, 121. For Catholic concerns over intermarriage and family planning, see Anderson, Interviews with Catholic priests, 8 Nov. 1933, General Interviews, Ethnic Study, ESV papers.

85. Anderson, *We Americans*, 259.

86. Ibid., 261–67.

87. Eduard C. Lindeman, Preface, *We Americans*, ix.

88. Hilda Wullen, Eugenics Research Association, to H. F. Perkins, 1 Nov. 1935, Perkins to Davenport, 18 Feb. 1936, Eugenics Research Association—Davenport, ESV papers. This exchange is the Perkinses' first communication with Davenport since 1932 and the first mention of ESV research since 1929. Perkins sent a paper on his adoption study but declined to attend the Eugenics Research Association annual meeting. See Laughlin and Davenport correspondence, March–May 1936, Eugenics Research Association, ESV papers.

89. Perkins, "Resumé of an Eleven Years Study," 25. For the investigation and closing of the Eugenics Record Office see Allen, "The Eugenics Record Office at Cold Spring Harbor," 251–54. For reviews of *We Americans*, see Robert K. Lamb, *New England Quarterly* (June 1938): 423–25; Gladys Bryson, *American Sociological Review* 3, no. 4 (1938): 597–98; Crane Brinton, *Saturday Review of Literature* 17 (Feb. 1938): 18.

90. Faculty Record Card, 1938, Faculty File, Henry F. Perkins, UVM Archives; Perkins to ESV Advisory Committee, 19 Oct. 1936. G. W. Bailey papers, UVM Archives.

91. H. F. Perkins, "Arnold and Allen: A Comparison and Contrast," *Vermont Alumnus* 17 (May 1938): 223–35. The speech was delivered at Ira Allen Chapel, 30 April 1938.

92. Perkins, "Arnold and Allen," 223–24. Perkins's framing of the question in terms of heredity, environment, and reaction had been promoted by Herbert Spencer Jennings in *The Biological Basis of Human Nature* (New York: W. W. Norton, 1930).

93. Perkins, "Arnold and Allen," 233.

94. Ibid.

95. H. F. Perkins, "Housing and the Next Generation," *Burlington Free Press*, Feb. 1939. Faculty File, Henry F. Perkins, UVM Archives; Anderson, *We Americans*, 241–42; American Eugenics Society, *A Eugenics Program for the United States* (New Haven: American Eugenics Society, 1935), 13. Promotion of birth control to reduce

procreation in large families living in poverty was the part of the new eugenic equation Perkins did not publicly pursue. See Mehler, "History of the American Eugenics Society," 271–82.

96. Perkins, "Resumé of an Eleven Years' Study," Guide to the Collection, ESV papers.

97. Ibid., 5–25; quotations on pp. 11, 13.

98. Vermont Children's Aid Society, Excerpts from the Report of the General Secretary, Oct. 1933, Oct. 1934, Oct. 1935, Special Collections, UVM Library.

99. Harold Bergman and Vonda Bergman, "These Are Our Own: The Vermont Children's Aid Society Comes of Age," *Vermonter: The State Magazine* 45 (Aug. 1940): 3.

100. Ibid., 6.

101. Dorothy Thompson, quoted in Bergman and Bergman, "These Are Our Own," 8. Thompson and her husband, Sinclair Lewis, owned an estate in Barnard, Vermont, which became a mecca for writers and political figures in the 1930s. As the first foreign correspondent to be expelled from Germany on Hitler's orders, a woman *Time* magazine recognized in 1939 as "the most influential woman in America next to Eleanor Roosevelt," her opinion of the Vermont Children's Aid Society was an honor.

102. Catherine Ashburner, "Shirley Farr," in *Those Intriguing, Indomitable, Vermont Women* (Vermont State Division of the AAUW, 1980), 41.

103. The Vermont Social Service Index (1934) was the outgrowth of files begun by L. Josephine Webster and the Vermont Department of Charities and Corrections in 1920. The state-administered index listed 11,311 individuals and three participating agencies in 1936. In 1946 over forty agencies participated, listing 50,797 persons. See Vermont Department of Public Welfare, *Biennial Reports of the Department of Public Welfare*, 1936, 11–12; 1938, 22; and 1946, 34–35.

104. Lillian M. Ainsworth, "Vermont's Feeble-Minded Problem," Report to T. C. Dale, Commissioner of Public Welfare, 1 January 1941, UVM Special Collections. For the development of psychiatric clinics and Ainsworth's role in the Board of Control of Mentally Deficient Persons, see Margaret B. Whittlesey, *The Vermont Conference of Social Welfare: The First Fifty Years, 1916–1966* (Burlington: The Conference), 8; Vermont Department of Public Welfare, *Biennial Report*, 1942, 6–8. For a contemporary discussion of the South Dakota eugenics program, see J. H. Craft, "The Effects of Sterilization as Shown by a Follow-Up Study in South Dakota," *Journal of Heredity* 27 (Oct. 1936): 379–87; Caroline Robinson, "Towards Curing Differential Births and Lowering Taxes, *Journal of Heredity*, 29 (June 1938): 230–34, and 29 (July 1938): 260–64.

105. E. Frieda Tracy et al., "What Mental Deficiency Means to the State of Vermont," typed MS containing four separate reports, ca. 1943, ESV since 1936, ESV papers. The report, prepared by eight social workers in the DPW, generally took the side of those dispossessed of their freedom and dignity through poverty and neglect by teachers, poormasters, and neighbors, yet they routinely buttressed their arguments with scholarly works by biologist-eugenicists R. A. Fisher and Herbert Spencer Jennings and Harvard anthropologist E. A. Hooton of nude posture photo fame.

106. "An Anthropological View of a Submarginal Culture, Or Some Vermont Families," in E. Frieda Tracy et al., "What Mental Deficiency Means to the State of Vermont," 10–18, quotation on p. 13.

107. "Save the Scrap," in E. Frieda Tracy et al., "What Mental Deficiency Means to the State of Vermont," 1–9, quotation on p. 9.

108. Tracy et al., "What Mental Deficiency Means to the State of Vermont," 5, 12, 22–26. For consistency of this report and Ainsworth's "Vermont's Feebleminded Problem" with the "new eugenics" of the AES, see AES, *American Eugenics Today* (New York: AES, 1939); Mehler, "History of the American Eugenics Society," 269–95.

109. Frederick C. Thorne, "Brandon State School," *Biennial Report of the Vermont Department of Public Welfare* (1946), 70. Dr. Thorne reported ten vasectomies and ten salpingectomies at Brandon during 1945–1946. For the consistency of Thorne's report with medical consensus and standard instituional practice of sterilization in the1940s, see Reilly, *Surgical Solution*, 129–39; Trent, *Inventing the Feeble Mind*, 222–24; Clarence J. Gamble, "Preventative Sterilization in 1948," *Journal of the American Medical Association* 141 (Nov. 1949): 773.

110. Thorne, "Brandon State School," 70. In 1951, Perkins cited the legal safeguards in the Vermont law in defense of allegations from the bishop of Burlington, who invoked Hitler's genocide of the Jews as the result of such a "so-called medical scientific procedure." "Dr. Harry Perkins Lauds Sterilization Law in Vt. But Bishop Ryan Condemns It," *Burlington Free Press*, 9 Oct. 1951.

111. "Perkins to Be Honored," *Burlington Free Press*, 26 April 1945; clipping, Faculty files, "Henry Farnham Perkins," UVM Archives.

112. Paul Amos Moody, "Frontiers of Knowledge in Biology," 22 Feb. 1945. Ira Allen Chapel, University of Vermont, Faculty File—"Paul A. Moody," UVM Archives. Paul Amos Moody, *Genetics of Man*, 2nd ed. (New York: W. W. Norton, 1975), dedication; H. J. Muller, "Progress and Prospects in Human Genetics," *American Journal of Human Genetics* 1 (Sept. 1949): 1–18. Muller rejected communism after Stalin's regime condemned genetics as "bourgeois, capitalist biology," liquidated all genetics research, and forced his Soviet colleagues into prison or exile. Muller's ideas surfaced in lectures by Moody in an interdisciplinary course on world problems in the early 1950s. See World Problems, Heredity East and West, Paul Moody papers, UVM Archives. Sociobiologists and evolutionary psychologists today have become fascinated with the ideas Moody expressed in 1945 and with hypothetical genes for "altruism." See, for example, Frank J. Sulloway, "Darwinian Virtues," review of *The Origins of Virtue: Human Instincts and the Evolution of Cooperation*, by Matt Ridley in *New York Review of Books* 65 (9 April 1998): 34–40.

113. H. F. Perkins, "The Vermont Commission on Country Life," *Vermont History* 23, no. 4 (1955): 335–40.

114. Ibid., 337.

115. Ibid., 338.

116. A Catholic adoption agency reported in 1948 the request of a sailor for a child. "With tears in his eyes," he told how his wife had been sterilized in one of the state institutions when she was fourteen and did not understand the implications when she had given her permission. "This girl was fit enough to be the wife of a sailor lad who serves his country . . . but was unfit to give that sailor lad a son . . . what master mind deprived this country of a future sailor boy?" *Vermont Catholic Review* 5 (Aug. 1945): 10; quoted in Loreno D'Agostino, *The History of Public Welfare in Vermont* (Winooski: St. Michael's College Press, 1948), 218–19.

Bibliography

Government and University Documents and Annual Reports

Ainsworth, Lillian M. "Vermont's Feeble-minded Problem." Report to T. C. Dale, Commissioner, Department of Public Welfare, 1 January 1941.

Buck v. Bell. 274 U.S. 200 (1927).

Governor's Commission of the Economic Future of Vermont. *Pathways to Prosperity: A Strategic Look.* Montpelier, Vt.: The Commission, 1989.

Governor's Commission on Vermont's Future. *Report of the Governor's Commission on Vermont's Future: Guidelines for Growth.* Montpelier, Vt.: The Commission, 1988.

Home for Destitute Children. *Charter and Rules and Regulations of the Home for Destitute Children at Burlington, Vermont.* Burlington, Vt.: Daily Times Printing House, 1866, 1892.

———. *Report of the Secretary and Treasurer of the Home for Destitute Children.* Burlington, Vt.: Home for Destitute Children, 1890–1899.

Laws of Vermont. 31st biennial sess. (1931):194–96. No. 174—An Act for Human Betterment by Voluntary Sterilization.

State of Vermont. *Vermont Statutes Annotated* (1987). Title 18, "Health," chap. 204, sects. 8705–16.

University of Vermont and the MCHV Health Choices Program. "Human Genetics: Navigating the New Frontier." George D. Aiken Lecture Series, 16 June 1994.

University of Vermont and State Agricultural College. *General Catalogue of the University of Vermont and State Agricultural College.* Burlington, Vt.: Free Press Association, 1895–1950.

Vermont. General Assembly. *Journal of the House of the State of Vermont. Journal of the Senate of the State of Vermont.* Montpelier: State of Vermont.

Vermont Children's Aid Society Annual Reports, 1920–1945.

Vermont Commission on Country Life. *Rural Vermont: A Program for the Future by Two Hundred Vermonters.* Burlington: Vermont Commission on Country Life, 1931.

Vermont Conference of Charities and Correction. *Proceedings of the Vermont Conference of Charities and Correction,* 1916–1917. Special Collections, University of Vermont Libary.

Vermont Conference of Social Work. *Proceedings of the Annual Conference of the Vermont Conference of Social Work,* 1918–1922; and *Reports of the Annual Meeting of the Vermont Conference of Social Work,* 1924–1936. (This organization was the Vermont Conference of Charities and Corrections in 1916–1918.)

Vermont Conference of Social Work Committee on Legislation. *Proposals for Improving Social Legislation in Vermont*. Burlington: Vermont Conference of Social Work, 1927.

Vermont Department of Public Welfare. *Biennial Reports of the Vermont Department of Public Welfare*. Montpelier: The Department, 1934–1946.

Vermont House and Senate Committee on Public Health Reports, 1927 and 1931, Vermont State Archives, Montpelier, Vermont.

Vermont Reports. In re Marcia R. 136:47–52. Oxford, N.H.: Equity Publishing Co., 1979.

Manuscript Collections

American Eugenics Society. Papers. American Philosophical Society Library, Philadelphia.

Bailey, Guy W. Papers. University of Vermont Archives, Burlington.

Davenport, C. B. Papers. American Philosophical Society Library, Philadelphia.

Huntington, Ellsworth. Papers. Manuscripts and Archives, Yale University Library, New Haven, Conn.

Eugenics Survey of Vermont and the Vermont Commission on Country Life. Papers. Public Records Office, Middlesex, Vt. This collection provides the most comprehensive record of the Eugenics Survey and the Vermont Commission on Country Life. The archive includes official and private communications of Harry Perkins and those associated with the Eugenics Survey, both within Vermont and with outside agencies; records of proposed projects, meetings, and publicity campaigns; raw data from particular studies; and a substantial portion of the "ESV Library," which Perkins created. The Guide to the Collection describes each investigation and contains a detailed inventory of the contents.

Faculty Files. University of Vermont Archives, Burlington.

Library Circulation Records. University of Vermont Archives, Burlington.

Moody, Paul A. Papers. University of Vermont Archives, Burlington.

Perkins, George H. Papers. University of Vermont Archives, Burlington.

Books, Articles, and Monographs

Aly, Götz, Peter Chroust, and Christian Pross. *Cleansing the Fatherland: Nazi Medicine and Race Hygiene*. Translated by Belinda Cooper. Baltimore: Johns Hopkins University Press, 1994.

Allen, Garland. *Life Science in the Twentieth Century*. New York: John Wiley, 1975.

———. *Thomas Hunt Morgan: The Man and His Science*. Princeton, N.J.: Princeton University Press, 1978.

———. "The Misuse of Biological Hierarchies: The American Eugenics Movement 1900–1940." *History and Philosophy of the Life Sciences* 5 (1984): 105–28.

———. "The Eugenics Record Office at Cold Spring Harbor, 1910–1940." *Osiris*, 2nd ser., 2 (1985): 225–64.

———. "Eugenics and American Social History, 1880–1950." *Genome* 31, no. 2 (1989): 885–89.

American Eugenics Society Board of Directors. *A Eugenics Program for the United States*. New Haven, Conn.: American Eugenics Society, 1935.

———. *American Eugenics Today*. New Haven, Conn.: American Eugenics Society, 1939.

Anderson, Elin L. *Selective Migration from Three Rural Towns and Its Significance. Fifth Annual Report of the Eugenics Survey of Vermont*. Burlington: Eugenics Survey of Vermont, 1931.

———. *We Americans: A Study of Cleavage in an American City*. Cambridge, Mass.: Harvard University Press, 1937.

———. *Rural Health and Social Policy*. Washington, D.C.: Michael M. Davis et al., 1951.

Anderson, Wilbert Lee. *The Country Town: A Study of Rural Evolution*. 1906. Reprint, New York: Arno Press, 1974.

Ann Arbor Science for the People Editorial Collective. *Biology as a Social Weapon*. Minneapolis: Burgess, 1977.

Appleby, Joyce, Lynn Hunt, and Margaret Jacob. *Telling the Truth About History*. New York: W. W. Norton, 1994.

Armstrong, Clarette P. "Toward a Democratic Eugenics." Review of *American Eugenics Today*, by the Board of Directors of the American Eugenics Society. *Journal of Heredity* 30 (April 1939): 163–65.

Ashburner, Catherine. "Shirley Farr." In *Those Intriguing, Indomitable, Vermont Women*. U.S.: Vermont State Division of the AAUW, 1980.

Bailey, Libert Hyde. *The Country Life Movement in the United States*. New York: Macmillan, 1911.

Barkan, Elazar. *The Retreat of Scientific Racism: Changing Concepts of Race in Britian and the United States between the World Wars*. Cambridge: Cambridge University Press, 1991.

———. "Reevaluating Progressive Eugenics: Herbert Spencer Jennings and the 1924 Immigration Legislation." *Journal of the History of Biology* 24 (spring 1991): 91–112.

Barker, David. "The Biology of Stupidity: Genetics, Eugenics and Mental Deficiency in the Inter-War Years." *British Journal for the History of Science* 22, no. 74 (1989): 347–75.

Bassett, T. D. Seymour. *A History of the Vermont Geological Surveys and State Geologists*. Burlington: Vermont Geological Survey, 1976.

Bergman, Harold, and Vonda Bergman. "These Are Our Own: The Vermont Children's Aid Society Comes of Age." *Vermonter* 45, no. 8 (1940): 183–88.

Bix, Amy Sue. "Experiences and Voices of Eugenics Field-Workers: 'Women's Work' in Biology." *Social Studies of Science* 27 (1997): 625–68.

Bliss, Laura, and Henry F. Perkins. "Fifteen Pairs of Twins: A Study of Similarities." *Eugenics* 2 (1929): 22–26.

Bower, William L. *The Country Life Movement in America*. Port Washington, N.Y.: Kennikat Press, 1974.

Bowler, Peter. *The Mendelian Revolution: The Emergence of Hereditarian Con-

cepts in Modern Science and Society. Baltimore: Johns Hopkins University Press, 1989.

————. "The Role of History of Science in the Understanding of Social Darwinism and Eugenics." *Impact of Science on Society* 40, no. 3 (1990): 273–78.

Brown, Dona L. *Inventing New England: Regional Tourism in the Nineteenth Century*. Washington, D.C.: Smithsonian Institution Press, 1995.

Bugbee, Sylvia J. "'Conservative Progessives': The Vermont AAUW and Its Drive for the Improvement of Rural Schools." Unpublished paper, Special Collections, University of Vermont Libraries, 1990.

Calloway, Colin G. "Surviving the Dark Ages: Vermont Abenakis during the Contact Period." *Vermont History* 58 (spring 1990): 70–81.

Campbell, Clarence G. "The Present Position of Eugenics." *Journal of Heredity* 24 (April 1933): 144–47.

————. "The Biological Foundations of Our Social Philosophy." *Eugenical News* 20, no. 2 (1935): 17–25.

Carnegie Foundation for the Advancement of Teaching. *A Study of Education in Vermont*. Bulletin no. 7. New York: The Foundation, 1914.

Caron, Joseph A. "'Biology' in the Life Sciences: A Historiographical Contribution." *History of Science* 26, no. 73 (1988): 223–68.

Castle, W. E. *Genetics and Eugenics: A Textbook for Students of Biology and a Reference Book for Animal and Plant Breeders*. Cambridge, Mass.: Harvard University Press, 1920.

Castle, William E., et al., eds. "William Keith Brooks: A Sketch of His Life by Some of His Former Pupils and Associates." *Journal of Experimental Zoology* 9 (1910): 1–52.

Clark, Ronald W. *The Survival of Charles Darwin: A Biography of a Man and an Idea*. New York: Random House, 1984.

Conklin, F. E., and Henry F. Perkins. "How Large Families Do Feebleminded Parents Have?" *Eugenical News* 13 (1928): 92–93.

Cook, O. F. "Human Hybrids in Virginia." Review of *Mongrel Virginians: The Win Tribe*, by Arthrur H. Estabrook and Ivan E. McDougle. *Journal of Heredity* 19 (March 1928): 115–18.

————. "Quenching Life on the Farm: How the Neglect of Eugenics Subverts Agriculture and Destroys Civilization." Review of *These Changing Times: A Story of Farm Progress during the First Quarter of the Twentieth Century*, by E. R. Eastman. *Journal of Heredity* 19 no. 10 (1928): 440–52.

Cook, Robert C. "Population Trends in Vermont." Review of *The Fifth Annual Report of the Eugenics Survey of Vermont: Selective Migration from Three Rural Towns and Its Significance*, by Elin Anderson. *Journal of Heredity* 23 (March 1932): 131–34.

————. "A Eugenics Program." Review of *A Eugenics Program for the United States*, by the Board of Directors of the American Eugenics Society. *Journal of Heredity* 27 (April 1936): 195–201.

Crow, James F. "Eugenics: Must It Be a Dirty Word?" Review of *In the Name of Eugenics: Genetics and the Uses of Human Heredity*, by Daniel J. Kevles. *Contemporary Psychology* 33 (January 1988): 10–12.

Cummings, Charles R. "The Inauguration As I Saw It." *Vermonter* 16 (November 1911): 371–94.

D'Agostino, Lorenzo. *The History of Public Welfare in Vermont*. Winooski: St. Michael's College Press, 1948.

Daniels, Robert D., ed. *The University of Vermont: The First Two Hundred Years*. Hanover, N.H.: University Press of New England, 1991.

Dann, Kevin. "The Purification of Vermont." *Vermont Affairs* 4 (summer/fall 1987).

———. "Gypsies in Vermont?" Paper presented at the Warren Sussman Memorial Graduate History Conference, Piscataway, N.J., April 1990.

———. "From Degeneration to Regeneration: The Eugenics Survey of Vermont, 1925–1936." *Vermont History* 59 (winter 1991): 5–29.

———. "The Natural Sciences and George Henry Perkins." *The University of Vermont: The First Two Hundred Years*. Edited by Robert V. Daniels. Hanover, N.H.: University Press of New England, 1991.

———. "The Pirate Family of Lake Champlain and Vermont Eugenics." Paper presented at Robert Hull Fleming Museum, Burlington, Vt., October 1995.

Davenport, Charles B. "Defects of Drafted Men." *Scientific Monthly* (January 1920): 5–25.

Degler, Carl N. *In Search of Human Nature: The Decline and Revival of Darwinism in American Social Thought*. New York: Oxford University Press, 1991.

Douglas, Mary. *How Institutions Think*. Syracuse, N.Y.: Syracuse University Press, 1986.

"Dr. Harry Perkins Lauds Sterilization Law in Vt. But Bishop Ryan Condemns It," *Burlington Free Press*, 9 October 1951.

Dubow, Saul. *Illicit Union: Scientific Racism in Modern South Africa*. Cambridge: Cambridge University Press, 1995.

Dunham, Paul C. *Population Trends and Their Implications on Government in Vermont*. Burlington, Vt.: Government Research Center, 1963.

———. *Vermont State Administrative Agencies*. Burlington: University of Vermont, Government Research Center, 1965.

Duster, Troy. *Backdoor to Eugenics*. New York: Routledge, 1990.

Eugenics Education Society. *Problems in Eugenics: Papers Communicated to the First International Eugenics Congress*. London: The Society, 1912.

Eugenics Survey of Vermont. *Second Annual Report of the Eugenics Survey of Vermont*. Burlington: Eugenics Survey of Vermont, 1928.

———. *Third Annual Report of the Eugenics Survey of Vermont*. Burlington: Eugenics Survey of Vermont, 1929.

———. *Fourth Annual Report of the Eugenics Survey of Vermont*. Burlington: Eugenics Survey of Vermont, 1930.

Farrall, Lyndsay Andrew. *The Origins and Growth of the English Eugenics Movement, 1865–1925*. New York: Garland Publishing Co., 1985.

Flint, K. R. B. *Poor Relief in Vermont*. Northfield, Vt.: Norwich University, 1916.

Foucault, Michel. *Madness and Civilization: A History of Insanity in the Age of Reason*. Translated by Richard Howard. 1961. Reprint, New York: Vintage Books, 1988.

———. *The History of Sexuality*. Vol. 1, *An Introduction*. Translated by Robert Hurley. 1976. Reprint, New York: Vintage Books, 1990.

———. *The Birth of the Clinic: An Archaeology of Medical Perception*. Translated by A. M. Sheridan Smith. 1963. Reprint, New York: Vintage Books, 1994.

Friedlander, Henry. *The Origins of Nazi Genocide: From Euthanasia to the Final So-lution*. Chapel Hill: University of North Carolina Press, 1995.

Galitzi, Christine Avghi. *A Study of Assimilation among the Roumanians in the United States*. New York: Columbia University Press, 1929.

Gallagher, Nancy. "Henry Farnham Perkins and the Eugenics Survey of Vermont." Master's thesis, University of Vermont, 1996.

Gamble, Clarence J. "Sterilizations of the Mentally Deficient in 1946." *American Journal of Mental Deficiency* 52 (1948): 375–78.

———. "Preventative Sterilization in 1948." *Journal of the American Medical Association* 141 (November 1949): 773.

Geddes, Patrick, and J. Arthur Thomson. *The Evolution of Sex*. Rev. Ed. London: Walter Scott, 1901.

Gill, Charles Otis, and Gifford Pinchot. *The Country Church: The Decline of Its Influence and the Remedy*. New York: Macmillan, 1913.

———. *Six Thousand Country Churches*. New York: Macmillan, 1920.

Goddard, Henry Herbert. *Feeblemindedness: Its Causes and Consequences*. New York: Macmillan, 1914.

Goldthwait, James Walter. "A Town That Has Gone Downhill." *Geographical Review* 17, no. 4 (1927): 528–52.

Gould, Stephen Jay. *The Mismeasure of Man*. New York: W. W. Norton, 1981.

Graff, Nancy Price, ed. *Celebrating Vermont: Myths and Realities* Hanover, N.H.: University Press of New England, 1991.

Guyer, Michael F. *Being Well-Born: An Introduction to Heredity and Eugenics*. Indianapolis: Bobbs-Merrill, 1927.

Haeckel, Ernst. *Last Words on Evolution: A Popular Retrospect and Summary*. 2nd ed. Translated by Joseph McCabe. London: A. Owen, 1906.

Hall, Max. *Harvard University Press: A History*. Cambridge, Mass.: Harvard University Press, 1986.

Haller, Mark H. *Eugenics: Hereditarian Attitudes in American Thought*. New Brunswick, N.J.: Rutgers University Press, 1963.

Hand, Samuel B., Jeffery Marshall, and Gregeroy D. Sanford. "Little Republics: The Structure of State Politics in Vermont, 1854–1920." *Vermont History* 53 (summer 1985): 141–66.

Harwood, Jonathan. "Genetics, Eugenics, and Evolution." *British Journal for the History of Science* 22, no. 74 (1989): 257–65.

Hasian, Marouf Arif, Jr. *The Rhetoric of Eugenics in Anglo-American Thought*. Athens: University of Georgia Press, 1997.

Haviland, William A., and Marjory W. Power. *The Original Vermonters: Native Inhabitants Past and Present*. Hanover, N.H.: University Press of New England, 1994.

Haycroft, John B. *Darwinism and Race Progress*. London: Sonneschein, 1895.

Hoffbeck, Steven R. "'Remember the Poor' (*Galations* 2:10): Poor Farms in Vermont." *Vermont History* 57 (fall 1989): 226–40.

Holmes, S. J. "'Facts of Heredity' for Race Conscious Germany." *Journal of Heredity* 25 (October 1934): 418–20.

———. *Human Genetics and Its Social Import*. New York: McGraw-Hill, 1936.

Huntington, Ellsworth, and the Directors of The American Eugenics Society. *Tomorrow's Children: The Goal of Eugenics*. New York: John Wiley & Sons, 1935.

Hubbard, Ruth, and Elijah Wald. *Exploding the Gene Myth: How Genetic Information Is Produced and Manipulated by Scientists, Physicians, Employers, Insurance Companies, Educators, and Law Enforcers*. Boston: Beacon Press, 1997.

Hutton, Patrick H. *History as an Art of Memory*. Hanover, N.H.: University Press of New England, 1993.

Huxley, Julian. "The Vital Importance of Eugenics." *Harpers* 163 (August 1931): 325–31.

―――. *New Bottles for New Wine*. New York: Harper and Brothers, 1957.

Huxley, Julian, A. C. Haddon, and A. M. Carr-Saunders. *We Europeans: A Survey of "Racial" Problems*. London: Jonathan Cape, 1935.

"Huxley Envisions the Eugenic Race." *New York Times*, 6 September 1937.

International Congress of Eugenics. *Eugenics, Genetics, and the Family*. Vol. 1 of *Scientific Papers of the Second International Congress of Eugenics*. Baltimore: Williams & Wilkins, 1923.

―――. *Eugenics in Race and State*. Vol. 2 of *Scientific Papers of the Second International Congress of Eugenics*. Baltimore: Williams & Wilkins, 1923.

―――. *A Decade of Progress in Eugenics: Scientific Papers of the Third International Congress of Eugenics*. Baltimore: Williams & Wilkins, 1934.

Jacobs, Margaret. *The Cultural Meaning of the Scientific Revolution*. New York: Alfred A Knopf, 1988.

Jordan, David Starr. "The Eugenics of War: Its Effect Principally on Heredity, and Wholly Pernicious—Military Training Cannot Compensate Because It Has No Effect on the Germ Plasm." *American Breeder's Magazine* 4, no. 3 (1913): 140–47.

Kempton, J. H. "Heredity, Environment and Human Fate." *Journal of Heredity* 21 (June 1930): 248–52.

―――. "Sterilization for Ten Million Americans." Review of *The Case for Sterilization*, by Leon F. Whitney. *Journal of Heredity* 25 (October 1934): 415–18.

Kevles, Daniel J. *In the Name of Eugenics: Genetics and the Uses of Human Heredity*. New York: Alfred A. Knopf, 1985.

Key, Wilhelmine E. *Heredity and Social Fitness: A Study of Differential Mating in a Pennsylvania Family*. Washington, D.C.: Carnegie Institute of Washington, 1920.

Klausen, Susanne Maria. "'For the Sake of the Race:' Eugenic Discourses in the *South African Medical Record*, 1903–1926, and the *Journal of the Medical Association of South Africa*, 1927–1931." Master's thesis, Queen's University, 1994.

Krause, Carol. *How Healthy Is Your Family Tree? A Complete Guide to Tracing Your Family's Medical and Behavioral History*. New York: Fireside, 1995.

Kraut, Alan M. *Silent Travelers: Germs, Genes, and the "Immigrant Menace."* New York: Basic Books, 1994.

Kuhl, Stefan. *The Nazi Connection: Eugenics, American Racism, and German National Socialism*. New York: Oxford University Press, 1994.

Larsen, Edward J. *Sex, Race, and Science: Eugenics in the Deep South*. Baltimore: Johns Hopkins University Press, 1995.

Lenz, Fritz. "Eugenics in Germany." *Journal of Heredity* 15 (March 1934): 223–31.

Lewontin, R. C. *Biology as Ideology: The Doctrine of DNA*. New York: HarperPerennial, 1993.

Lifton, Robert Jay. *The Nazi Doctors: Medical Killing and the Psychology of German National Socialism.* New York: Basic Books, 1986.

Locy, William Albert. *Biology and Its Makers.* New York: H. Holt, 1908.

"Looks to Rural Life to Preserve Race," *New York Times,* 5 June 1932: 29.

Lovett, Laura. "Speaking in the Vernacular: Florence Sherbon and the Promotion of the Family Ideal." Paper presented to the Organization of American Historians, Indianapolis, April 1998.

Lubove, Roy. *The Professional Altruist: The Emergence of Social Work as a Career.* New York: Atheneum, 1975.

Ludmerer, Kenneth M. *Genetics and American Society: A Historical Appraisal.* Baltimore: Johns Hopkins University Press, 1972.

Lund, John M. "Vermont Nativism: William Paul Dillingham and the U.S. Immigration Legislation." *Vermont History* 63 (winter 1995): 15–29.

Lynd, Robert S., and Helen Merrell Lynd. *Middletown: A Study in Contemporary American Culture.* New York: Harcourt, Brace, & Co., 1929.

Martin, Luther, et al. "Eugenics, Genetics, Ethics, and Art." Symposium, Robert Hull Fleming Museum, Burlington, Vt., 1995.

Mayr, Ernst. *Toward a New Philosophy of Biology: Observations of an Evolutionist.* Cambridge, Mass.: Harvard University Press, 1988.

McCullough, Dennis M. "W. K. Brooks's Role in the History of American Biology." *Journal of the History of Biology* 2 (1969): 411–38.

McLaren, Angus. *Our Own Master Race: Eugenics in Canada, 1885–1945.* Toronto: McClelland and Stewart, 1990.

Mehler, Barry Alan. "A History of the American Eugenics Society." Ph.D. dissertation, University of Illinois, Urbana-Champagn, 1988.

Moody, John. "The Native American Legacy." *Always in Season: Folk Art and Traditional Culture in Vermont.* Ed. June C. Beck. Montpelier: Vermont Council on the Arts, 1982.

———. "The Impact of Eugenics on Abenaki Families in Vermont." Paper presented to the New England American Studies Association, Providence, R.I., April 1996.

Moody, Paul Amos. *Genetics of Man.* 2nd ed. New York: W. W. Norton, 1975.

Moore, James R. *The Post-Darwinian Controversies: A Study of the Protestant Struggle to Come to Terms with Darwin in Great Britian and America, 1870–1900.* Cambridge: Cambridge University Press, 1979.

Muller, H. J. *Out of the Night: A Biologist's View of the Future.* New York: Vanguard Press, 1935; New York: Garland Publishing Co., 1985.

———. "Progress and Prospects in Human Genetics." *American Journal of Human Genetics* 1, no. 1 (1949): 1–18.

Neill, Maudean. *Fiery Crosses in the Green Mountains: The Story of the Ku Klux Klan in Vermont.* Randolph Center, Vt.: Greenhills Books, 1989.

Newman, Horatio Hackett. *Readings in Evolution, Genetics, and Eugenics.* Chicago: University of Chicago Press, 1921.

———. *Evolution, Genetics, and Eugenics.* 3rd ed. New York: Greenwood, 1932.

Oatman, Michael. "Long Shadows: Henry Perkins and the Eugenics Survey of Vermont." Exhibit at Robert Hull Fleming Museum, Fall, 1995.

Odem, Mary E. *Delinquent Daughters: Protecting and Policing Adolescent Female*

Sexuality in the United States, 1885–1920. Chapel Hill: University of North Carolina Press, 1995.

Osborne, Frederick. *Preface to Eugenics.* New York: Harper & Bros., 1951.

———. *The Future of Human Heredity: An Introduction to Eugenics in Modern Society.* New York: Weybright & Talley, 1968.

———. "History of the American Eugenics Society." *Social Biology* 21, no. 2 (1974): 115–26.

Paul, Diane B. "Eugenics and the Left." *Journal of the History of Ideas* 45 (October–December 1984): 567–90.

———. "Eugenic Anxieties, Social Realities, and Political Choices." In *The Politics of Western Science.* Edited by Margaret C. Jacob. Atlantic Highlands, N.J.: Humanities Press International, 1994.

———. *Controlling Human Heredity: 1865 to the Present.* Atlantic Highlands, N.J.: Humanities Press, 1995.

Paul, Diane, and Harnish G. Spencer. "The Hidden Science of Eugenics." *Nature* 374 (23 March 1995): 302–4.

Pearl, Raymond. "The Biology of Superiority." *American Mercury* 12, no. 47 (1927): 257–66.

Pearson, Karl. *Eugenics Laboratory Lecture Series: The Francis Galton Laboratory for National Eugenics.* London: Dulace, 1909; New York: Garland Publishing Co., 1985.

Perkins, Henry F. "The Development of Gonionema Murbachii." *Proceedings of the Academy of Natural Sciences of Philadelphia* 54 (December 1902): 750–90.

———. *Notes on the Medusae of the Western Atlantic.* Publication 102. Washington, D.C.: Carnegie Institute of Washington, 1905.

———. "Review of Eugenics in Vermont." *Vermont Review* (September–October 1926): 56–59.

———. *Lessons from a Eugenical Survey of Vermont. First Annual Report.* Burlington: Eugenics Survey of Vermont, 1927.

———. "Hereditary Factors in Rural Communities." *Eugenics* 3 (August 1930). (Reprint in Special Collections, Bailey Howe Library)

———. "Make Haste Slowly." *Journal of Heredity* 24 (April 1933): 148–49.

———. "Contributory Factors in Eugenics in a Rural State." In *A Decade of Progress in Eugenics: Scientific Papers of the Third International Congress of Eugenics.* Baltimore: Williams & Wilkins, 1934.

———. "Arnold and Allen: A Comparison and a Contrast." *Vermont Alumnus* 17 (May 1938): 223–32.

———. "A Resumé of an Eleven Years' Study, 1925–1936." Unpublished manuscript, ca. 1938, in the Guide to the Collection of the Eugenics Survey of Vermont manuscript collection. Public Records Office, Middlesex, Vermont.

———. "The Vermont Commission on Country Life." *Vermont History* 23 (October 1955): 335–40.

Pernick, Martin S. *The Black Stork: Eugenics and the Death of "Defective" Babies in American Medicine and Motion Pictures since 1915.* New York: Oxford University Press, 1996.

———. "Eugenics and Public Health in American History." *American Journal of Public Health* 87, no. 11 (1997): 1767–72.

Perrin, Noel. "The Two Faces of Vermont." *Vermont Life* 19 (winter 1964): 31–35.

Pickens, Donald K. *Eugenics and the Progressives.* Nashville, Tenn.: Vanderbilt University Press, 1968.

Popenoe, Paul. "Feeblemindedness Today. A Review of Some Recent Publications on the Subject." *Journal of Heredity* 21 (October 1930): 421–31.

———. "The German Sterilization Law." *Journal of Heredity* 25 (June 1935): 257–60.

Popenoe, Paul, and Roswell H. Johnson. *Applied Eugenics.* New York: Macmillan, 1922.

Potash, P. Jeffrey. "Deficiencies in Our Past." *Vermont History* 59 (fall 1991): 212–26.

Rafter, Nicole Hahn. *White Trash: The Eugenic Family Studies, 1877–1919.* Boston: Northeastern University Press, 1988.

Rebek, Andrea. "The Selling of Vermont: From Agriculture to Tourism, 1860–1910." *Vermont History* 44 (winter 1976): 14–27.

Reilly, Philip R. *The Surgical Solution: A History of Involuntary Sterilization in the United States.* Baltimore: Johns Hopkins University Press, 1991.

Robinson, Caroline. "Towards Curing Differential Births and Lowering Taxes." *Journal of Heredity* 27 (Oct. 1938): 230–34; 29 (July 1938): 260–264.

Robinson, Rowland E. *Vermont: A Study in Independence.* Boston: Houghton, Mifflin & Co., 1892.

Robinson, William J. *Woman: Her Sex and Love Life.* New York: Eugenics Publishing Co., 1927.

Roll-Hansen, Nils. "The Progress of Eugenics: Growth of Knowledge and Change in Ideology." *History of Science* 26, no. 73 (1988): 295–331.

———. "Genetics and the Eugenics Movement in Scandinavia." *British Journal for the History of Science* 22 (September 1989): 335–46.

———. "Eugenic Sterilization: A Preliminary Comparison of the Scandinavian Experience to That of Germany." *Genome* 31, no. 2 (1989): 890–95.

Roosevelt, Theodore. "Twisted Eugenics." *Outlook* 106 (3 January 1914): 30–34.

Rosenberg, Charles E. *No Other Gods: On Science and American Social Thought.* Baltimore: Johns Hopkins University Press, 1976.

Roth, Randolph. "Why Are We Still Vermonters? Vermont's Identity Crisis and the Founding of the Vermont Historical Society." *Vermont History* 59 (fall 1991): 197–211.

Rubin, Herman. *Eugenics and Sex Harmony: The Sexes, Their Relations, and Problems.* New York: Elliott, 1933.

Ryan, Patrick. J. "Unnatural Selection: Intelligence Testing, Eugenics, and American Political Cultures." *Journal of Social History* 30, no. 3 (1997): 669–85.

Shapiro, Henry D. *Appalachia on Our Mind: The Southern Mountains and Mountaineers in the American Consciousness, 1870–1920.* Chapel Hill: University of North Carolina Press, 1978.

Sherman, Michael. "'The Spanish Influenza' in Vermont, 1918–1919." Paper presented to Research-in-Progress Seminar, Center for Research on Vermont, Burlington, October 1994.

Sherman, Michael, and Jennie Veersteg, eds. *We Vermonters: Perspectives on the Past.* Montpelier, Vt.: Capital Press, 1992.

Taylor, Henry C. "The Vermont Commission on Country Life." *Journal of Farm Economics* 12, no. 1 (1930): 164–73.

Thomson, J. Arthur. *The Science of Life: An Outline of the History of Biology and Its Recent Advances*. Chicago: Herbert Stone, 1899.

————. *Heredity*. New York: G. P. Putnam's Sons, 1908.

Trent, James W., Jr. *Inventing the Feeble Mind: A History of Mental Retardation in the United States*. Berkeley: University of California Press, 1994.

True, Marshall. "Middle Class Women and Civic Improvement in Burlington, 1865–1890." *Vermont History* 56 (spring 1988): 112–27.

Webster, Josephine. *The Vermont Children's Aid Society, Inc.: The First Fifteen Years, 1919–1934*. Burlington, Vt.: Queen City Printers, 1964.

Weindling, Paul. "The 'Sonderweg' of German Eugenics: Nationalism and Scientific Internationalism." *British Journal for the History of Science* 22, no. 74 (1989): 321–33.

Weingart, Peter. "Politics of Heredity: Germany, 1900–1940, a Brief Overview." *Genome* 31, no. 2 (1989): 896–97.

Wessel, Bessie Bloom. *An Ethnic Survey of Woonsocket, Rhode Island*. Chicago: University of Chicago Press, 1931.

Westman, Jack C. *Licensing Parents: Can We Prevent Child Abuse and Neglect?* New York: Insight Books, 1994.

Whiting, P. W. "Communist Eugenics." Review of *Out of the Night: A Biologist's View of the Future*, by H. J. Muller. *Journal of Heredity* 27 (March 1936): 132–35.

Whittlesey, Margaret B. *The Vermont Conference of Social Welfare: The First Fifty Years, 1916–1966*. Burlington: Vermont Conference of Social Welfare, 1966.

Wiggam, Albert Edward. *The Next Age of Man*. Indianapolis: Bobbs-Merrill, 1927.

Wilson, Harold Fisher. *The Hill Country of Northern New England: Its Social and Economic History in the Nineteenth and Twentieth Centuries*. Montpelier: Vermont Historical Society, 1947.

Wright, Lawrence. *Twins: And What They Tell Us about Who We Are*. New York: J. Wiley, 1997.

Index